"*Sarah is not the 'rah-r* [...] *style. She knows, just like* [...] *......... ....y .... in that approach. Sarah is much more considered, much more caring, much gentler yet deeper at the same time. And all of that comes with massive traction – and hence positive, life-changing moments for everyone who happens to have the privilege of sharing her insights.*"

Paul Dunn
Chairman of B1G1, four-time TEDx speaker, Singapore

"*Sarah has been my most influential life adviser. She is a brilliant teacher and helps me make sense of concepts that no one else has been able to explain. This book is the starting point.*"

Matt Murphy
Managing Partner, MPR Group

"*I have read many books in pursuit of finding purpose and becoming a better version of myself. Sarah's ability to help you focus on what matters most, based on real experience, is what enables her to make a significant impact on the lives she touches.*"

Lisa Morris,
Global Employee Experience Consulting Practice Leader

"*This should be a part of every leader's toolkit. Sarah automatically brings you perspective and the ability to see the bigger picture, which in our frenzied world, where the key focus is often very short-term, can be invaluable.*"

Jill McMillan
Director of Leadership and Development, Bank of America

"*She lets you get out of being totally in your head and brings you back to life with levity. It's getting into your heart. It's getting into the soul of who you really are without you really realising she's doing it. It's magical.*"

Jacqueline Shaulis
Founder, Awesome Enterprises LLC

ENERGY On Demand:
Master your personal energy and never burn out

by Sarah McCrum

Energy On Demand:
Master your personal energy and never burn out
Author: Sarah McCrum

ISBN: 978-1-84914-054-6
© Sarah McCrum 2016

www.sarahmccrum.com
sarah@sarahmccrum.com

Editing by: Alex Mitchell | www.authorsupportservices.com
Cover by: Julia Dyer
Design by: Laren Graterol | laren.graterol@gmail.com
Illustrations by: whiteboardgirl at www.fiverr.com
Printed and bound by: Completely Novel

This book is dedicated to the people who are too busy to read it.

Acknowledgements

As I wrote this book it became simpler and simpler, which made me happy as I worked out the essence of what to share with you. This simplicity was only possible because of the people who have helped me over many years by pushing me again and again to clarify who I am, what I'm doing and what's important to me.

I'd like to thank the people who taught and trained me, especially my Chinese Masters, Zhixing Wang and Aiping Wang, and Ian Mussman of Alpha Gamma Brain. Your knowledge has no price and deserves to be shared more widely.

Three organisations have played a special role in the last few years with their training programs. The Entrepreneur Institute started me off with iLab. Key Person of Influence gave me a massive step up – I wouldn't have written a book without you and Andrew Griffiths. And most recently Seth Godin's altMBA program pushed me further than anything else to figure out what I'm doing with my life. So thank you to all of you.

Another group of people plays a very special role in my life – my clients. I won't mention you by name, but you are the lifeblood of my learning. I feel so lucky to be able to say that I love every minute of working with each one of you. It's immensely humbling to be the person who gets to hear your inner world in such detail and to share your journey towards a more joyful, purposeful and fulfilling life. This book is founded on my experiences with all of you.

Thank you to Anna Sanchez, who is unfailingly willing to listen to my ideas and ask the gentlest yet most probing questions, and to Alex Mitchell who was willing to start editing the book with two days' notice and who kept me on track.

My final and biggest thank you goes to my husband, Niko. You give me so much support, appreciation and love. I am truly grateful.

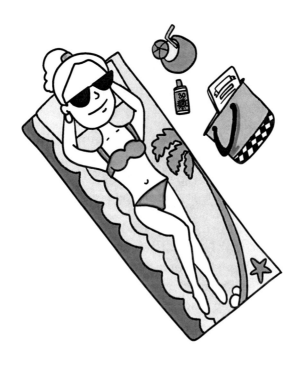

Preface

I was lying on the beach on an island in Greece, fast asleep. Every now and then I woke up, had a swim, and fell asleep again. When I was hungry I'd find something to eat and then I slept again. I went on like this for several weeks. I had no energy.

I was 26 years old and I'd burnt out after my third year as a teacher in an English boarding school. I still remember the feeling. I had no will, no wish to do anything except sleep and soak up the Mediterranean sun.

And then one day I felt a spark. My energy started to return. Soon my motivation came back and I found myself ready to work - so I started the cycle all over again.

It all fell apart a few years later, six months after my younger sister died of a brain tumour. This time I needed professional help and I had my first acupuncture session. Miraculously, I felt absolutely fine within an hour. It was my introduction to the Chinese world of energy and I was hooked.

Soon afterwards, I began 22 years of training with two Chinese Masters, in London, Croatia and New Zealand. This changed the way I thought, felt and viewed the world, and I've lived and breathed the language, philosophy and practice of energy ever since.

In 2000 I created a business in London called The Energy Bank. My team and I taught leaders from companies like Virgin Media, Bank of America and Dow Jones, along with many small business owners, how to have more energy and get amazing business results by being relaxed and at peace.

Since 2012 I've been living in Australia, coaching CEOs and leaders. It's obvious to me that a lot of business problems could be solved easily if more people knew how to take care of their personal energy.

We've largely overlooked this topic in the West, to the extent that we find it normal to abuse our energy every day. A few advanced companies, like Google, are beginning to realise how important energy is, and science is slowly waking up too, but I couldn't wait any longer.

After working with so many people and seeing so many improvements in health and wellbeing, productivity and performance, business development and finance, as well as family relationships and simple things like happiness and inner peace, I had to start sharing this knowledge more widely. This book is the first step.

Contents

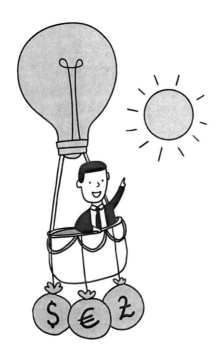

Introduction

This book is for you if you want more energy.

It's for you if you have very little time, work far too hard, never stop thinking and know that this is not sustainable.

You are the kind of person I've worked with for the last 20 years and I want to share my experience with you.

I'm not going to give you the facts and figures about why you should do something about your energy or what the latest science says about it. If you don't have enough energy you know you need to do something about it, and you don't need to waste any time filling up your head with more to think about. One thing is for sure – your head is already too full and you're craving relief and inner peace.

So I invite you to take this book, and its accompanying online course, as a solution to the problem of not having enough energy. I'm going to give you a very easy way to solve the problem – it may even seem too easy and hard to believe at times. And I'm going to ask you to trust the process I will introduce and simply follow it so you can find out for yourself how it works.

How to read this book

The book introduces six keys to having more energy. It starts with the simplest, most practical key, and becomes gradually richer and deeper as you go.

For each key I have given you a few things to do or reflect on that will change your energy. You shouldn't try to do everything in the book right away. Although it's short, there's enough material in here to stimulate several years of exploration.

I recommend you approach the book as follows:

Start by reading 'The 5 Day Energy Charge', 'What is Energy' and the chapter called 'Relax'.

Then begin the 5 Day Energy Charge. This is an online course that will teach you in a very practical way how to get more energy by relaxing every day for 5 days. It's included free of charge with the book.

If you don't have enough energy, your first priority is to learn how to relax.

This is not the way you might usually relax (in front of the TV or with a glass of wine or something stronger), but a simple, special method that will give you energy.

Once you're settled and have started the 5 Day Energy Charge, come back to the book and read some more. If you come to a chapter that appeals to you, practise one of the suggested activities.

You're aiming to make the activities part of your lifestyle, so it's best to take one at a time and practise it for a minimum of 30 days until it's so familiar that it has become a habit. Then you can move on and incorporate another practice if you want.

If you don't resonate with any of the suggestions, just ignore them. Do what feels right, and you'll naturally and intuitively begin to create more energy in your life.

Energy On Demand

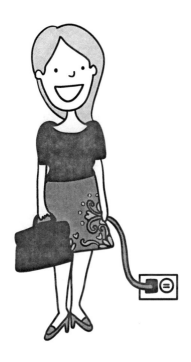

The 5 Day Energy Charge

The 5 Day Energy Charge is an online course, designed to help you increase your energy in a short period of time and experience benefit as soon as possible.

It consists of 5 guided audio relaxations, during which you will be led into a state of deep relaxation. You can listen to each of them as many times as you want. This is the simplest and fastest way of receiving more energy and making a difference to your life here and now.

You may think relaxation sounds like the opposite of what you need if you're short of energy, but I assure you that it works. This is where you need to trust the process and just do it. You'll discover why later.

All you need for the online course is a computer or mobile device, some earphones and a comfortable chair, preferably in a quiet location (but don't worry if the chair or location aren't perfectly ideal – the process will still work).

- Go to this link: http://courses.sarahmccrum.com/bundles/ energy-on-demand
- Click the pink button as if to buy the course.
- On the next page enter the following coupon code to reduce the price to zero: **energy**
- Complete the 'purchase' (checking that the coupon has been applied and the price is zero) and you can get started.
- Follow the instructions and relax every day for 5 days without fail.
- If you miss a day, it doesn't matter. Just start again and aim to do 5 days straight.
- When you sign up for the 5 Day Energy Charge you will also get access to Energy On Demand - Online Course. This is a multi-media course made from the contents of this book.

Go ahead and sign up for the 5 Day Energy Charge now.

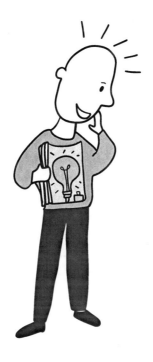

What is energy?

One morning you wake up full of joy. You jump out of bed, ready for the day. You're happy. You're relaxed. You're going to enjoy your day and you feel great. You're full of energy.

A couple of days later you wake up and you don't even want to open your eyes. It's hard to crawl out of bed. You need a cup of coffee before you can move. You drag yourself through the first couple of hours of the day dreading what you've got to do, and wondering how you're going to get through until evening.

There's only one fundamental difference between these two scenarios – your energy.

When you're full of energy, life feels easy, comfortable and relaxed. You enjoy it, you feel present and connected and you can perform at any level you want.

When your energy level is low, you don't feel like doing anything. Everything feels like a struggle. You don't enjoy your day and you have very little motivation.

Energy is your 'get up and go'. It's your physical capability, your mental ability, your emotional state and your spirit. It's the essence and sum total of who you are.

Energy is what gives you your capacity and motivation for life. It's the life force that flows through you and keeps you going every day. It determines your performance, your impact on the world and your quality of life.

> *Energy is your 'get up and go'. It's your physical capability, your mental ability, your emotional state and your spirit.*

Why is energy important?

Imagine you have one hour in which to make an important business decision.

If your energy is so low that you're lying in bed sick, hardly able to think, in pain and feeling terrible, you're unlikely to make any decision at all.

If you're at work, your desk is a mess, you have a pile of jobs you need to do, there are people needing your help, you're trying to keep everybody happy and you're feeling stretched in every direction, you're likely to make a rushed decision which may not be very effective.

On the other hand, if you have a team that's running smoothly and you're able to take some time to reflect first, you could make a decision worth tens or hundreds of thousands of dollars in that hour. You could make a single phone call with great presence of mind and clarity and get an outcome that changes the course of your business.

If you're running a world-class business at the top of your game, you could make a decision that passes millions of dollars across the world, bringing opportunity to millions of people because you have the capacity to think and act on a global scale.

Your energy, and the energy of the people you attract to work with you, is the essence of your business. The quality, performance and scale of your business are all determined by your energy.

If you want to be more successful, you need to understand that working hard to grow your business while exhausting your energy supply is a short-term strategy that leads to disappointment.

If, however, you learn how to protect and grow your energy as you grow your business, your success will be sustainable and you'll get to enjoy the benefits for a long time to come.

> *Energy determines your performance, your impact on the world and your quality of life.*

Most people have very little idea what energy really is. You take it for granted most of your life, only discovering how much you need it if you begin to run out of it. But what does energy really do?

At a business level, it makes you more efficient, more effective and better at performing. You can focus more effectively, your mind becomes clearer and you have better concentration. For example, if a challenge comes up, while other people are reacting defensively, you go instantly into a relaxed, clear state. You know exactly what needs to be done.

You don't make a big fuss about circumstances because you don't need to command attention through noise and excitement. Instead, you command attention through your energy, quietly and calmly moving pieces and influencing people to do what needs to be done.

When you have more energy you have more enthusiasm, enjoyment and fun. You're like a magnet – people want to work with you and you attract more support, more opportunities and more business.

As you expand your energy, you also get on better with other people. Your relationships become easier and you feel more comfortable with yourself and others.

Having more energy unblocks problems. You find solutions far more easily. You get better ideas and the right people cross your path at the right time.

You also have more energy for your family, social life and weekends. If you really take care of your vitality, you don't need to crash for the first few days of your holidays because you're already in good energetic shape.

This all sounds rather magical, and the honest truth is that sometimes it feels rather magical. It's the opposite of the hard work we're used to, and it can be difficult to believe that life can be so much easier and less demanding just by having more energy.

How to have more energy

Following, in brief, are the six keys to getting more energy. Each will be fully explored in its own chapter later on. You may already be doing some of these things, and you don't need to master them all – at least not yet. Sometimes a small tweak can free up a lot of energy for you.

The first key, relaxation, is the master key to all the others. If you want to employ just one tactic, this is the most efficient, effective and powerful of them all. It's the one you need as a foundation for all the others, so it's most definitely the place to start.

1. Relax

At its simplest level there's only one thing you need to do to have more energy. Learn how to relax.

Those words are easy to say but can be hard to do if you're busy. Relaxing feels like the one thing you don't have time for. And if you do have some time, your mind is usually running so fast that there's no relaxation in it.

Yet that's the classic sign of someone who desperately needs to learn how to relax.

2. Balance your energy

If you're lacking energy or at risk of burning out, you've developed an imbalance. The tricky thing is that some of your good habits may be making you more unbalanced than you realise, especially if you pride yourself on your performance.

> *At its simplest level there's only one thing you need to do to have more energy. Learn how to relax.*

But the good news is that when you learn how to rebalance your energy your performance improves at the same time. It becomes easier to achieve at a higher level and keep going in the long-term.

3. Recharge your energy

Most busy people treat themselves like a rechargeable battery they never have time to fully charge. Our regular ways of recharging through food, exercise and sleep don't seem to be up to the job any more.

That's why it's necessary to learn new ways of recharging your energy, over and above what you're already doing. This is simple and satisfying and it makes a big difference to your quality of life.

4. Sustain your energy

Once you're relaxed, have a bit more balance and are able to recharge your energy whenever you need to, it's time to talk about sustainability. There's no point in getting into shape and then letting it all go again.

It's a lot easier to improve your lifestyle by now, because you have the energy to do it, and the magic is that some of it will happen effortlessly.

5. Expand your energy

Your energy is a valuable asset and a major key to your satisfaction in life. It's at the heart of who you are and what you want from life.

> *Energy is your most precious resource. It responds well to being treasured, loved and invested in.*

When you know how to expand your energy as you evolve, this will support you in achieving your greater goals and connecting with your true potential and uniqueness.

6. Supercharge your energy

Some people are so peaceful and connected that they can do great things, but they're rarely born that way. They've learned techniques which help them access a more powerful source of energy than the rest of us.

When you do the same things you will have access to the same source they do. This is where your energy practice goes deeper and makes a more profound difference to your life.

Every step on this journey gives you more energy than you currently have access to. It's a simple process and each of the steps is easy to learn. It takes practice and there are downs as well as ups, but you're used to that. It's no different from anything else you've ever learned.

If you want a satisfying experience I recommend you leave impatience at the door and give yourself time. Energy is an important enough resource to be worth investing in. The returns are far greater than the time you put in, and it takes remarkably little effort.

Alex Blyth is Founder and Managing Director of Mega Adventure Group, which runs an adventure park on Sentosa Island in Singapore, another in Adelaide, Australia, and several other attractions in Singapore. When I first met him he was thinking about starting a business but hadn't written the plan yet.

I found the corporate world constricting and conformist and I'd always promised myself that I would never end up in that kind of environment. If I was going to go into business by myself then it should be fun, challenging and entertaining - no two days the same.

In 2007 I met you and we started having a discussion about energy, source, the power of the universe and the laws of attraction. All these elements seemed to flow automatically into the business I was building.

There's no reason why I should've achieved what I've achieved. To give you some idea, after five to six years, we'll have ten million dollars in turnover and it's getting larger. We've expanded into Australia. We have six different businesses now.

That wasn't achieved through spreadsheets, analysis and over-thinking things. It was achieved, I believe, largely by having the right approach, the right attitude and by building a foundation which you amongst others have helped me to establish. A foundation of ethics based around relationships, trust, loyalty, faith, humour - all these have allowed me to attract the right people and build something that's more about the energy than the numbers.

Yes, it's about humour. It's about fun. It's about a wonderful sense of what we call enthused desire, glorious delight. It's about building an environment people enjoy being in, whether that's a client, a person who's working alongside us or a supplier. It's about having fun, enjoying each other's company and building rapport and a sense of energy.

If you'd have put me in these shoes ten or fifteen years ago, I'm not sure I would've been able to manage that. Now I seem to manage it effortlessly and I don't say that with any sense of arrogance or superiority. It's fallen into place and the reason is because I've trusted and relaxed.

Relaxation has become a cornerstone of success. It's something you get better and better at. I now couldn't function without stopping everyday and relaxing.

When you change your energy, you change your life. Working on your energy affects every area of your life because it affects you, and you are the central player in your life. Energy work integrates your personal and business life and allows you to feel as if you're one person living one life, rather than wearing several different hats in different roles.

Energy is your most precious resource. It responds well to being treasured, loved and invested in, not wasted, spent or thrown away. If you care for your energy in the same way that you care for your most loved person or possession, you'll find yourself on a path to a life filled with enjoyment and purpose.

Energy is...

- effortless
- simple
- at your pace
- a little every day
- and it takes patience
- _____
- _____
- _____
- _____
- _____

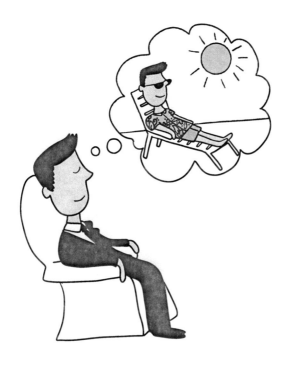

1
Relax

Let's take a look now at the first and most fundamental key to working with your energy – relaxation.

Energy flows constantly through your system, providing life force to all the tissues and organs of your body. A healthy person has a balanced flow of energy coming in and going out. You become unhealthy when you lose this balance.

The simplest and most common way you reduce or block your flow of energy is by becoming tense. Tensing up physically contracts your muscles, and this constricts the energy channels, or meridians.

The meridians, according to Chinese medicine and acupuncture, are subtle energetic channels that run through the body. Each is associated with a different organ, and collectively they carry your vital life force. When you become tense the meridians shrink, and less energy is able to flow through them.

It's normal to become tense from time to time when you experience challenges or pressures. This doesn't do any harm as long as you're able to relax again and open up your meridians. When you do, more energy will flow through your system and you'll regain your balance.

Problems arise when you repeatedly or constantly tense up and restrict the flow of energy through the body. There are different ways this might happen.

> *When you're relaxed, you're not tense. It's that simple.*

1.   You're generally tense for an extended period of time. This restricts your overall flow of energy so you gradually experience having less and less of it. All your organs and bodily systems receive less energy, so your wellbeing and eventually your health deteriorate.

2. You tense up a particular part of your body regularly. This restricts the flow of energy to the meridians that pass through that part of the body. In turn, the organs that are supplied by those meridians receive less energy than they require and become weaker. This gradually affects you emotionally and physically, making you feel unwell or blocked.

What's the remedy for all this tension? It's to be relaxed. When you're relaxed, you're not tense. It's that simple.

But there's a problem. Many people think they know how to relax but they're still tense. I hear this all the time. "I know how to relax.

I can watch television or read a book or have a glass of wine." Yes, these are popular ways of relaxing, but they're not very effective in preventing tension in the longer term.

You can come home from work every day and sit in front of the television for a few hours. And while you may feel relaxed by the time you go to bed, that feeling will likely not last when you get to work the next day.

Or you can go away on holiday and do very little for a fortnight. But how long will it be before you're stressed again when you return? For most people it's not very long.

Luckily, there is a way to make the feeling of relaxation stick around even after you're done actively relaxing.

Energy relaxation is a way of relaxing that actually gives you energy. It's different from purely physical relaxation. It's somewhat similar to meditation, but it's easier and has additional energetic benefits.

> *When you're relaxed, happy and at peace, you naturally attract people, money, business and opportunities.*

Some business people grow nervous when I talk about relaxation. They're worried they'll no longer be able to perform if they relax because they need to keep themselves constantly amped up to stay on top of business.

The problem is that this is a short-term approach. If you keep yourself pumped up all the time, it's like trying to fly a fighter jet without ever stopping to refuel or perform maintenance. You won't be able to sustain that energy level in the long term.

When you learn to relax, you'll discover that you naturally attract business without having to chase it. One of the things many people notice when they first start relaxing is that, even in the first weeks, they draw new business to themselves without making any effort at all. Sometimes they'll even close a deal that had previously been problematic.

As you open up and become more relaxed, you'll experience that people want to work with you more. They appear to be attracted to your presence. When you're relaxed, happy and at peace, you naturally attract people, money, business, opportunity and everything else you want.

Long term benefit

While the short term benefits can be significant, the real difference occurs when you take time to relax every day over six months, a year, two years or even longer. It's been 27 years for me and things continue to improve. There's no end to the need for deep relaxation in our lives.

If you keep going your health improves continuously. Your relationships gradually get better and better, and the same thing happens to your business. The more relaxed you are the happier you are, and the better business you're able to do. Things are better for you, better for your team, better for your clients and better for your other stakeholders.

How to relax for more energy

The essence of energy relaxation is doing nothing, but it's doing nothing in a special kind of way. Very often when we think we're doing nothing, we're really doing something. We're thinking, unconsciously squeezing and releasing muscles, or trying to escape from life by reading a book or watching TV.

Energy relaxation is a way of doing nothing that makes you more alive. You stop being occupied with all the physical and material stuff that's right in your face and you do absolutely nothing at all.

You take a little time just to be. You don't try to be somebody in particular, but just let yourself exist as you are. When you take that time to be and to do nothing, after a little while everything starts to change.

To begin with, you may find yourself very occupied with thoughts, but gradually you notice yourself letting go of some of that. You start to see and feel things differently. If you go a little further, you'll discover that through doing nothing, you gain energy and you feel more alive.

Energy relaxation is a way for you to stop getting in the way of your life and let it function as it's designed to do. Things become a great deal easier.

> *Energy relaxation is a way of doing nothing that makes you more alive.*

A simple way to get started is deliberately to set aside some time to do nothing.

Sit down somewhere – maybe somewhere nice, but not so engaging that you get really involved in the place. See what happens when you don't do anything at all. Stop thinking about work. Stop trying to solve all your problems and stop being preoccupied with anything. Stop worrying and just let life be life for a little while.

That is the heart of relaxation.

The beauty of it is that the process becomes an upward spiral. When you relax, you gradually let go of tension and receive more energy. As more energy starts to flow through your system, you feel better. As you feel better, you relax more and receive even more energy. The more energy you have, the more relaxed you feel.

A step by step method to relax quickly

It's often hard to find time to sit and do nothing until you're relaxed, so it's good to have a faster method that relaxes you almost instantly.

For this method, you'll need about 20 minutes when you're not going to be disturbed. Switch off your mobile phone, close the door and give yourself a break.

Read the instructions below so you know what to expect, but keep in mind that learning how to relax from a piece of writing is a bit like learning how to ski from a book – in other words, not easy. So please don't expect to be able to relax easily just because you've read the method. It's a skill, not a mental activity, and it takes some practice.

This is a great time to start the 5 Day Energy Charge, where you'll learn to relax and receive energy as you listen to the audio recordings (see the link in the '5 Day Energy Charge' section on page 5). It's the easiest and most efficient way to learn.

Position

Sit in a comfortable chair with your back well supported. It's good if your neck and head are also supported so you can lean back and let go (but this is not essential). Reclining chairs are fine.

Point your face slightly upwards as if you are looking at the morning sun.

Put your hands lightly in your lap, not touching each other.

Stretch your legs out loosely in front of you with both feet on the ground.

Close your eyes.

Let your whole body relax.

Alternatively, you can lie on your back with your arms by your side (but sitting is recommended because it's easy to fall asleep when you're lying down).

Step 1 - Relax

Let your full weight sink down into the chair. Imagine you're melting into it.

Breathe gently into your stomach and lower belly. You should feel your belly expanding as you breathe in and contracting as you breathe out.

Relax your feet by allowing them to soften and expand a little. Feel the relaxation in your feet for a little while.

Then relax the different parts of your body in the same way, feeling them soften and expand as you turn your attention to them.

From your feet, move up to your legs and relax them.

Relax your hips, then your stomach and lower back in the same way.

Relax your chest and upper back.

Relax your shoulders, arms and hands.

Finally, relax your neck, jaw and head.

As you progressively relax, your body may become warmer and feel softer.

Step 2 - Empty Your Mind

Relax your face and your forehead.

Start to empty your mind of thoughts.

If thoughts come to you, treat them as if they're very unimportant so there's no need to engage with them.

Just let them go.

Forget whatever you've been doing today.

Forget any problems or worries.

Forget what you're going to be doing later or tomorrow.

Imagine you're listening to the silence in your mind, not the noise.

Step 3 - Wait

There's no need to concentrate or focus on anything.

Just sit and wait.

Relax and wait.

Wait some more, doing nothing.

You may start to feel some energy in your body. There are many different ways you might experience this (described below).

Whatever you feel, it's important simply to relax.

Enjoy.

Many different feelings and experiences can occur while you're relaxing. These are the sensations of energy flow. They can be a bit different from regular physical sensations. You may experience one or more of the following:

A warm current flowing through the body

Waves of energy through the body

Feeling tingly all over or in certain parts of the body

A warm pleasant feeling

A soft warm casing around your body

Cool air flowing over you

Seeing bright colours with closed eyes

Seeing a light shining inside or outside of your body

Visions and dreamlike states

A feeling of floating or rocking.

Sometimes you drop into a state of emptiness where everything goes dark and still. It's a very nice place where there's nothing going on at all – no thinking, no inner activity. This is a very healing space. You completely let go of all your worries and preoccupations and receive a lot of fresh energy.

The further you go, the more kinds of experiences you'll have. Sometimes they're beautiful, sometimes ordinary. The main thing about all of these experiences is that they're passing and they change. Don't get hooked by or hung up on them. Sometimes they repeat, sometimes not. The only goal here is to spend time relaxing.

David Smith is a geologist and leader in the mining industry. Over a 4-month period he built up a habit of relaxing daily and this is what he said:

For me, relaxation is the key to performing and making good decisions. I've been able to be more effective with less effort. This sense of efficiency and productivity is not in the traditional sense of me getting more done, but of more happening in my presence. More gets done and I have to do less personally.

The things that I have on my list for the day that I think, in a left-brain sort of way, really need to get accomplished, seem to get taken care of with much less effort than before. Either conditions change and they no longer need to be done, resources show up that take care of them - for example somebody else does them - or I'm able to accomplish them with a relaxed sense of flow and less work than I anticipated. That has given me an even deeper sense of relaxation that everything is getting taken care of and that I have support.

As a result my sense of scope has expanded hugely. By that I mean the size of the opportunities that I'm involved in have gotten much bigger than they've ever been before and I'm comfortable at that level. I'm in bigger deals and playing in a larger field with a deeper sense of comfort than I used to have in smaller arenas. That sense of expansion has been huge. I know that's a direct result of relaxing.

Questions

How often should I relax?

It's best to relax every day so you build up a habit of feeling relaxed. You should do it once a day (or more if you like).

What's the best time to relax?

I recommend you relax first thing in the morning if you possibly can, because this sets up your energy for the whole day. It's a great way to put yourself in a state of flow.

It can be good to relax in the evening if you have trouble sleeping. You may fall asleep during the relaxation, which is fine.

It can be very useful to relax at lunch time, even just for ten minutes if you're very busy, because this will set up your energy for the afternoon so you don't have that mid-afternoon slump.

It can also be good to relax when you come home from work, even if it's only for five or ten minutes, just to let go of the day and give yourself the energy you need for your family and social life.

Any other time of day is also fine.

There's no good excuse for not taking some time to relax. If you're super busy you can relax on the fly while you're picking up the kids, sitting in a meeting, standing in the lift or working at your computer. But it's much more beneficial to make the time to sit down and relax deliberately when there's nothing else going on.

Take your cue from Gandhi, who said, "I have so much to accomplish today that I must meditate for two hours instead of one".

What happens if I forget?

It's very important to realise that when you first start learning to relax you'll probably forget to keep doing it. Most people do after a few days or a few weeks. Some people forget after the first day.

To get started, it's easier to set yourself a target to do it every day for a set period of time so you can build up a habit and experience the benefits.

I recommend you insist on relaxing every day for 5 days. If you miss a day, start again. Keep going until you've achieved 5 days in a row. This is why I've included the 5 Day Energy Charge with this book. That makes it much easier to keep track of your relaxation sessions.

Then you can expand to 30 days – or be brave and commit to 100 days. Start again if you miss a day. A good way to prevent forgetting is to have an accountability partner or do it as a group challenge so you can support and remind each other. Check out the 30 Day Energy Challenge on my website, *www.sarahmccrum.com*.

> *The quiet you're looking for is internal, not external.*

What if I can't find anywhere quiet to relax?

It's not critical to be in a quiet place. I often relax in trains, on planes, in waiting rooms and anywhere else I can get a few minutes to be calm. The quiet you're looking for is internal, not external.

My benchmark is that I want to be relaxed on a busy London roundabout during rush hour or when everything's going wrong at work. I can practise that anywhere – and so can you.

Why couldn't I relax well today?

The goal of relaxation is simply to show up every day. Sometimes it's going to feel horrible. Sometimes it's going to feel wonderful. You don't have to feel relaxed every time you practise. In fact, you won't. Sometimes you'll think all the time. Sometimes you'll want to stay there forever because it feels so beautiful. The only significant outcome is that you will gradually feel better and better over time.

It's very, very important to understand that you can't do it right and you can't do it wrong. It's not about right and wrong. It's simply about doing it and learning and growing from what you experience.

> *It's very, very important to understand that you can't do it right and you can't do it wrong.*

What should I do if my mind is constantly busy when I'm relaxing?

Sometimes people say, "I just don't feel like I'm doing it right because my mind is chattering through the whole relaxation".

Please don't judge your relaxation. Sometimes it feels really good and your mind clears. This is nice and can make you feel that you're doing it right. But other times you'll feel you're not relaxing well. Your mind may be busy or you may remain tense throughout. That doesn't mean it wasn't a good relaxation. You still get the benefit even if you don't consciously feel it.

The point is, relaxation comes in different forms. The so-called 'bad' ones are good, and so are the good ones, of course. The general principle with relaxation is that it's always good – so keep doing it.

Why do I sometimes feel uncomfortable after relaxing?

In addition to all those positive signs of energy flow mentioned earlier, energy also has a kind of 'detoxing' effect.

When you relax, you receive a lot of life force and it starts to clean out the blocked and toxic energy in your body that has been stored there for a very long time. You're likely to experience some uncomfortable effects from this.

It's very important to be aware of this phenomenon because when it hits you, you can easily become confused. You may feel as though you've got a cold or flu for a few days. You may feel achy in your body. You may feel symptoms of an old sickness coming up. These are all good signs that your body is detoxing.

You may experience many different kinds of physical symptoms. You might suddenly feel itchy. You might feel pain in some part of your body that you don't normally have. Sometimes you can get some odd energetic feelings

> *The general principle with relaxation is that it's always good – so keep doing it.*

inside your body that are very difficult to describe.

If you have an existing health problem, you might feel the symptoms getting worse for a while. This is usually the hardest thing to deal with. You're supposed to be getting better but you feel as though you're getting worse. Just imagine that you're spraying a jet hose through your body, cleaning out a lot of rubbish. If you were already ill, there was definitely rubbish in there. Your increased symptoms are a sign that the rubbish is being cleaned out. It's like cleaning a dirty house. You make a big mess while you're doing it, but the final result is good.

You may also have a period during which you feel more emotional than usual. You might experience an emotional outburst or you might go through strong waves of emotion.

It's very common for people who are depressed or emotionally sensitive to experience waves of emotion for quite a long period. When a wave hits you it can feel terrible. And when you're detoxing through relaxation some of those waves can feel worse than normal, but after each one passes you will feel much better than you've felt in a long time. That's one of the things to look forward to.

There are many different detoxing effects. The general principle is that the negative feelings you experience are old energy being released from your body. It's energy you no longer need. The older it is, the more unpleasant it might feel to release. If you've been very tense for a long time, you can expect quite a lot of releasing. There's a lot of energy stuck in your system. But the end result will be worth it.

> *Trust the process.*

When will I start detoxing? I have an important meeting and I need to be in good shape for it.

It hits different people at different times. Some people start detoxing almost as soon as they start to learn to relax. Some people don't experience anything for months.

In my experience, if you have an important meeting you'll be fine. Somehow your body knows what's on your agenda and it manages the timing for you.

Why do I seem to be so unstable?

If you've become very out of balance and your body (or your life) is rebalancing through relaxation, you may find yourself swinging from one emotion to another, sometimes feeling wildly off course. It will feel as though life is pushing you all over the place. This may also happen with physical symptoms.

It's uncomfortable, but remember that you're healing. Every time you feel out of balance there's a natural healing process going on.

The key is to let go of trying to control everything and let nature do its job. It's far more intelligent than your limited mind and will rebalance you automatically if you allow it.

One of the simplest ways to learn to let go of control is by relaxing even more. The more you learn to relax, the more you're able to feel the energy that's flowing into you, and then you have much more of an idea about how to manage yourself on a day to day basis.

This is particularly hard for control freaks. All I can say is to trust the process. Trust nature, because the more you do so, the more balance you'll find in your life.

Will I feel sleepy when I relax?

Most people don't feel sleepy when they finish relaxing. They tend to feel full of energy and more alive.

If you're somebody who thinks a lot you may find that the only way you can switch off is to fall asleep while relaxing. Sometimes you feel as if you're partially asleep, but still slightly awake. It's like being in a deep place where you can dimly hear the outside world but you're so far away from it that it no longer affects you. This will happen naturally and it's fine.

If you're really, really exhausted and you've been pushing yourself beyond your limits for a long time, you may feel very tired for a few days. This is a sign that you need to get more sleep. Take it as a warning. Make sure you relax every day and find some way to catch up on the sleep that you've been missing.

Can relaxation help me with challenges in my work?

There are some specific situations where it's really useful to relax, especially if you find them challenging or you want to be at your best.

You can relax before a presentation, an important phone call (maybe for just two minutes or so), a meeting, a networking event, an interview, a date or anything that makes you feel nervous.

One woman told me how much difference relaxation has made in her life. "When I forget to do my relaxation, I feel like I want to kill my husband, but if I do the relaxation, I just feel like I want to massage him and I understand why he's so tense and stressed. I'm a completely different person."

The magic

Sometimes things happen in a way that seems magical when you're relaxed and have more energy.

Business shows up unexpectedly; your partner seems to change and become more positive; your team is more cooperative even though you didn't do anything special; support comes just when you need it even though you didn't ask for it.

This magical effect will gradually increase as you become more relaxed, but you never know when and you can't force it. If you try to make it happen it never works, but if you're happy, relaxed and at peace, you have a natural force of attraction, and sometimes things happen beautifully and magically for no obvious reason.

So don't expect it – but enjoy it when it happens!

If you want to relax...

- let go
- just be
- do nothing
- empty your mind
- change will happen
- _____
- _____
- _____
- _____
- _____

Energy On Demand

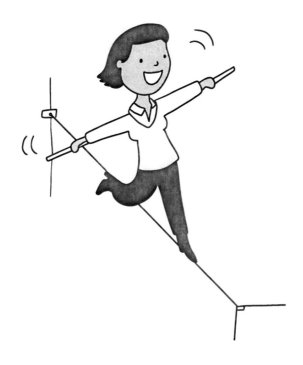

2

Balance your energy

In business and in life, balance means you can steer a path through your many challenges whilst you retain clarity of mind. You have the ability to make wise decisions and there's space in your life for periods of peak performance as well as times of reflection and recovery.

Energy balance is a state of being poised between positive and negative, or what the Chinese call yang and yin, both of which always exist. If you have a best, you have a worst. If you have good, you have bad. If you have up, you have down. Everything comes in opposites. If you try to deny one side exclusively in favour of the other, you become unbalanced.

Balance is not static – it's very dynamic. It's like somebody on a tightrope; if you watch them, you'll see that they're never absolutely still. They're wobbling slightly all the time to either side of their balance point.

In the same way, energetic balance is something to perpetually aim towards, not a state of perfection you'll ever reach.

Feeling balanced gives you an inner steadiness and peacefulness and the ability to move forward. If you become very unbalanced, you stop moving forward because you have to work so hard to maintain yourself where you are.

In today's business world of ultra-connectivity, it's easy to live a very unbalanced life. For example, it can be all about productivity and getting as much done as possible without creating quieter or more reflective times when you slow down and get some perspective.

If you're always trying to be your best – inspired, positive and on top – you have to push yourself constantly. You try so hard to get ahead that you end up attempting to control everything so it doesn't all collapse. What tends to emerge is a state of anxiety, nervousness and feeling perpetually wired. You find yourself constantly stressed. The ultimate result is that you're very likely to burn out.

Or you might take the opposite approach by slowing down, but in a resigned sort of way. Everything's going too fast for you, so you feel you can't cope and you disengage. You become resistant and bored, and this eventually leads to extreme dissatisfaction, depression or a sense that your life is stuck, going nowhere.

Each of these scenarios reflects an inner state of imbalance and each ultimately leads to some kind of breakdown, whether you burn out or get sick. This is nature's way of pushing you to rebalance. You have to come back into balance to be able to move forward again.

How to balance your energy

Here are two ways to rebalance your energy. The first is based on the Chinese principle of yin and yang energy. When they are in balance within you, and in your life, your energy will feel balanced.

The second is grounding. If you're ungrounded you'll tend to feel very unbalanced. I give you several different grounding exercises. Just pick one that feels right for you.

Balance your yang and yin energy

Yang and yin energy are the positive and negative aspects of energy that need to be balanced.

Yang describes anything that is more active, directed or defined. A great deal of business activity is yang, including striving, performing and achieving goals.

Feeling balanced gives you an inner steadiness and the ability to move forward. It is something to aim towards, not a state of perfection you'll ever reach.

Yin describes a more inclusive, softer, gentler, more expansive energy. Caring, nurturing and receiving are all yin activities. They tend to be harder to measure – the softer skills – but just as important.

If you tend to be too yang (the overdrive type), you need to put some yin time into your week. This is a powerful way to maintain balance and prevent yourself from burning out.

Some yin activities:

· daydreaming

· lolling about in the ocean (not swimming to get fit or surfing to prove yourself)

- spending time in the garden, picking a few flowers, appreciating the beauty and wandering in a purposeless way, just enjoying yourself
- going for a wandering kind of walk, smelling the roses, stopping to appreciate nature, walking slowly and immersing yourself in beauty
- having a long hot bath with a couple of handfuls of epsom salts (good if you can't go to the ocean) and letting yourself go without thinking
- doing nothing, just sitting quietly with no intention except to be
- reading poetry (but not other types of reading) and appreciating its beauty.

> *If you tend to be too yang you need to put some yin time into your week, and vice versa.*

If you tend to be too yin (the caring sensitive type who doesn't accomplish things), then doing some more yang activities is really good for you.

Some yang activities:

- create a to do list and get it done
- do any achievable, measurable task
- go for a walk and stride out to get your circulation moving
- go to the gym
- clean up your desk, the shed or an area of the house
- plant an area of the garden and complete the task.

Note: if you've been working under pressure for many years and you've burnt out, you may find yourself feeling depressed and slow, unable to get anything done. This means you may look like a yin type, but it comes from having been too yang.

In this case it's important to allow yourself time to recover and rebalance naturally. Yin activities are good for you. You're being yin to balance out the excess yang. At a certain point you will start to recover your balance and become more active again.

Ground your energy

When you become imbalanced you can also become ungrounded. This feels as though all of your energy is in your head, or that your brain is very busy all the time. You can also feel as though you're floating through life without ever putting your feet down on the ground.

In contrast, grounded people are practical and get things done without getting over-excited about them. Here are several different grounding exercises.

1. This first exercise is very simple. You can do it anywhere, even at your desk.

   · Sit on a comfortable chair with both feet on the ground.

   · Close your eyes and breathe gently down into your stomach and lower belly.

   · Let the weight of your body sink down into the chair. Your body may start to feel heavy. You may feel a sensation of heaviness going down through your feet and into the ground. Your energy is grounding, dropping down.

   · Let it keep dropping down further and further for several minutes.

   · At a certain point you may feel as though some energy is coming up from the earth back into you. Then you're grounded. The down and up movements are balanced.

- This is a subtle feeling so don't worry if you can't feel anything. It may take some practice. Just do it anyway.

2. Walk barefoot on the beach, the grass or a wooden floor. Make sure you don't get cold feet.

3. Walk slowly, imagining that your feet are sinking into the ground with each step. Keep doing this for at least five minutes, or longer if you have time. You may find yourself speeding up naturally after a while. If you practise regularly the sensation of your feet sinking into the ground becomes more and more real, giving you a tangible feeling of energy. It's unusual and can make you feel very relaxed, energised, or both.

4. Do something practical, physical or manual. Gardening, cleaning, fixing things, making things, creating.

5. Connect with your belly. Breathe gently into your lower belly. There's an energy centre about two horizontal fingers width below your navel which the Chinese call the Dantian. This is also your physical centre of gravity. As you breathe, allow your lower belly to expand. Feel that the Dantian area just below your navel is expanding, as though there's a balloon inside that's gently being blown up or a ball of energy that's gently expanding. The ball of energy may feel as though it is expanding beyond your physical body. Do this for five minutes, or longer if you can.

6. Connect with your heart. This is a good technique to make you feel softer, more open and more receptive (more yin). Place your hands gently on the centre of your chest, one on top of the other. There's another energy centre here called the heart centre. Sit quietly and breathe into your heart centre. Allow your mind to quiet down. You may feel your heart beating, or some pressure or other sensations in your heart. Take a few minutes simply to feel without thinking about it. Whatever happens is okay.

Jeremy Harris is a partner at Gill McKerrow, an accounting firm in Brisbane, Australia, who was looking for more energy when I first met him.

I was facing some struggles that were taking a toll – extremely low energy, anger and frustration, and a lack of quality time with my family. My business was not growing the way I wanted, despite it being the main focus of my life.

Instead of peace and calmness there was frustration and anger, and most of that was directed at myself, my own imperfections and mistakes.

Now I feel like almost nothing can ruffle me or rock the boat. Things come up where the boat will rock but it doesn't take much to steady it again because that inner peace and calmness can really take over if I just get out of the way and let it.

Paradoxically, I have learnt that I gain more control of my life when I let go. I have found balance. The energy and focus that are required to perform well in my work are in abundant supply and easy to connect to. I make decisions more easily now, without the guilt and overthinking that used to accompany them. Now, once a decision is made, it is done. When it's time to go home and connect with my family, that same energy is available to fuel my connection to them.

One of the most remarkable transformations I have experienced is the change in the people around me. My family is more calm, and I have a more open relationship with my business partner than I had before. More than anything, kindness and peace are what will bring the best results in both business and family. Both, to a degree, are about leadership and at the same time about being very present and engaged.

I am learning not to dwell on my mistakes. The phrase 'It is what it is' helps me to not overthink situations. It may have been a mistake, but big or small there is a reason situations occur the way they do. The point is that I need to learn from my experiences, positive or negative, big or small, professional or personal.

Realising that I need to learn and then let things go has been a monumental change for me. Learning to speak more productively and openly to other people in my life has been very valuable. My communication is much more productive now, and is more buoyant for the other people involved.

I also speak better to myself. I treat myself better. I used to speak to myself in a way that I would be ashamed of if I was observing myself doing it. If I was a little boy on the receiving end of the way I was speaking to myself I would feel terrible.

As a result of all of this, I am having more fun with my business which has led to a more consistent flow of new client inquiries, and new clients coming on board that I would have thought impossible in the past. Of course this has resulted in increased financial flow, which is incredible.

Questions

What can I do about negative self-talk?

One really big thing to watch out for is negative inner talk and guilt.

If you tend to be too yang, you probably have an inner voice that says things like, "I should be doing something. I should be busy. There's so much to do. There's so much I've got to get done. This is ridiculous. This is such a waste of time. I'm not achieving anything here. Look at me. I'm just thinking all the time anyway, so there's no point in doing this because it's not going to work. I'd be better off doing something useful." Your mind will go on and on like this.

If you tend to be too yin and you're trying to get things done or take action, there will be negative talk as well, and it will go something like this: "This is a complete waste of time. There's no point in doing anything. Everything I do goes wrong. Everything I do is a failure. This isn't worth it. Even if I do this, it's not going to make any difference. Nothing makes any difference to me."

It's extremely important to take no notice of the negative voices and simply do what you need to do to rebalance your energy. The purpose of the activity is what's important, not the voices that go on inside your mind. They are simply filling up space. Nothing they say is actually true.

It helps to be kind to them as though they are misguided children. You're not trying to eliminate or destroy them, because that tends to make them even stronger. Give them some love and then just keep doing what you need to do.

> *It's much more valuable to strive for excellence than perfection.*

How can I do this properly? I don't ever seem to find true balance in my life.

You may be trying to be perfect. Perfectionism almost always leads you perfectly in the wrong direction. If you keep on trying so hard to be perfect, you might find you end up in completely the wrong place.

When you're driving you're almost never perfectly on track. You're making constant tiny adjustments to your direction. If you go a little bit too far one way you automatically correct yourself because otherwise you'd find yourself driving off the side or into the middle of the road.

The honest truth is you don't know exactly how to get to wherever you're going. Even if you have a very clear goal, you don't know what the challenges are going to be along the way. It's much more valuable to strive for excellence than perfection, and then you can make constant corrections to get closer and closer to what you want. This will keep you more balanced – but never perfect. So stop trying so hard to be that way and enjoy the ride instead.

The beauty

The beautiful thing about rebalancing your energy is that at a certain point you'll stop thinking about how wobbly you were. You'll feel fine and you may not even realise it. Business will be going smoothly and it will feel like it was always smooth.

Life starts to feel as though this is how it was always supposed to be. It's so natural you might wonder why it ever felt hard. You feel more powerful and more at ease than you have for a very long time. And life is beginning to be more enjoyable, too. It's a beautiful feeling.

Keys to balance your energy.

- Let go to gain control.
- Energetic balance is a journey.
- Balance creates clarity.
- Balance = calm and peace.
- _____
- _____
- _____
- _____
- _____

Energy On Demand

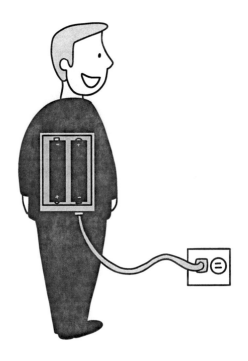

3

Recharge your energy

When I was growing up I only remember one type of battery. It was like the cheap ones today that don't hold their charge for long. When alkaline batteries came onto the market they seemed very expensive and over the top. I couldn't imagine why we would need them.

We tend to treat ourselves like cheap rechargeable batteries and expect that by sleeping, eating, exercising and having some fun, we'll keep our batteries fully charged.

Traditionally that may have been enough because we weren't demanding so much of ourselves. But in the society we live in now and with the kind of demands we place on ourselves, sleep, food, and exercise are no longer enough for most of us to maintain our energy at the level we want. That's the reason why we need to learn how to recharge our energy.

If you keep your energy well charged, and recharge it on time, you experience consistent performance over a sustained period. You have a stable supply of energy that you can rely on when you face demanding challenges, and you can generate additional energy quickly and efficiently when you need it.

If you don't know how to recharge your energy well, you become stressed and drained more easily. Very often the first part of your life to be affected is your sleep. If you're not sleeping well you lose even more energy, and this will gradually affect all your other ways of recharging. When you're tired you tend to eat less well, exercise less and have less fun.

> *If you keep your energy well charged, you experience consistent performance over a sustained period.*

The obvious response is to boost your energy another way, so you may turn to caffeine. This will give you a kick, but if you always use stimulants to wake yourself up and get through the day, the wiring you'd normally use to recharge yourself becomes lazy because you don't use it anymore.

Then you may start to need an artificial system to relax as well. You drink coffee to keep yourself going and then you need alcohol to relax, sleeping pills to sleep or recreational drugs to have fun.

Now you have a double dose of artificial substances replacing natural functions. That's not a great solution. Unfortunately it's the cultural solution. There are very, very few people I come across who don't drink coffee to give themselves energy, but it's easy to get energy without coffee once you know how.

How to recharge your energy

Even if you're relaxing every day, your energy levels will fluctuate all the time. Sometimes this is caused by external factors that have nothing to do with you, and sometimes it's because of your activities. If you're very busy you may need to top up your energy more than usual. If you're under a lot of emotional pressure, such as during major life events, you will also find your energy level dipping and it will need additional support.

You may already know of some activities that help you recharge. Perhaps it's playing golf, going swimming, having some time alone, having a massage or meeting a particular friend. Here are some other ways to recharge that are applicable to everyone and frequently overlooked during times of stress.

Sleep

A basic way to recharge your energy is to sleep well. If you have problems sleeping, take some time to relax before you go to sleep. You can also listen to a guided relaxation in the middle of the night if you find yourself awake. Very often it will send you to sleep again. If not, it will still recharge you so that you don't feel tired during the day.

Often people who wake up in the middle of the night spend many hours thinking. It's very important to break that habit. You can fool yourself into imagining you're solving problems by thinking about things, but you're not. Once you learn to relax instead of ruminating, solutions will show up far more quickly.

It helps to have regular sleep patterns. That means always going to bed and getting up at the same time, as far as possible.

It's better to go to bed earlier and get up earlier if you can. The Chinese say that the universe cleans the energy of the day between 11.00pm and 3.00am. This makes sense if you imagine going out into a city at 10.00 or 11.00 at night. The atmosphere can be quite negative. It feels clogged up and heavy. If you go to the same place at 3.00 in the morning, it feels much fresher.

Being in bed and asleep by 11.00pm is a very positive thing. It keeps you out of the way of the negative energy that's being removed from the atmosphere.

Take time off

Another way to recharge your energy, which is fairly obvious yet often overlooked, is simply to take some time off work and stop thinking about it. If you have a lot of responsibility you may need to schedule time with your partner or your family, time alone and time for enjoyment. And by the way, there's no point taking time off work to be glued to your mobile phone and thinking constantly.

It's important to get away from digital life on a regular basis. Leave the mobile phone behind, close the computer and get out into nature – whatever it takes to switch off. It's ideal to be digital-free for a while every day, especially before you sleep.

And take holidays.

It's so easy to imagine that if you just keep working you'll get more done. But once you start to understand more about energy, you'll discover that you often get more done when you stop working. You can spend all day thinking about a problem when all you really need to do is take a short walk and clear your mind. Do that, and the solution will come to you without any effort at all.

If you have trouble giving yourself permission to take time off, put it into your calendar. Make sure your appointments with yourself are as sacrosanct as your most important meetings.

Enjoyment

Enjoyment is an incredibly important part of the energy cycle. In fact, if you enjoyed more of your life you probably wouldn't need a book like this at all. Enjoyment is the essence of energy.

Having a good time with friends, doing things you enjoy or taking some time to enjoy doing very little – these are all important things you may have lost touch with. If you're very driven it becomes so important to get things done that you can forget how to enjoy yourself.

When you enjoy yourself, you relax naturally. That's why it energises you. Give yourself permission to do things you love.

Be present

This is a way of recharging your energy while you're busy. It takes some inner focus, but it's very rewarding and can completely change the flow of your day.

> *Enjoyment is the essence of energy.*

Being present means having a clear mind and remaining 'in the moment' rather than being distracted by thoughts related to the past or the future. If you're in a meeting, simply listen and speak when you need to and let go of everything else that has nothing to do with the meeting.

If you're working at your computer, reserve some energy to remain present. This means staying very relaxed and focused on what you're doing without being intense. You keep your head clear, so there are no extraneous thoughts crowding in.

You can't do this on autopilot. It takes a little awareness to stay present, but if you practise it regularly you'll get better and better at it. If you make sure you're relaxing at the same time, you'll find yourself receiving energy as you work rather than spending it.

Fiona Ballantyne is a senior audit partner at a global accounting and consulting firm. She was experiencing problems because of long term stress from her job. She describes the changes that resulted from a program of daily relaxation.

I was experiencing many health concerns that were affecting the quality of my work and my life. High blood pressure, hormonal imbalances, adrenal fatigue, anxiety and nervousness.

These resulted in me finding myself unable to get through the day, feeling ill equipped to manage the stress and challenges that I faced. This affected the quality of my relationships, both personal and professional, my leadership capability and the level of fulfilment I got from my work.

I saw medical professionals, but they were unable to find a root cause for any of these symptoms. Their solution was to prescribe medication for the symptoms, which seemed to me like a very poor approach long term. I also saw a naturopath, who prescribed supplementation, but I did not see the improvement that I was seeking. What's more, I experienced side effects from the supplementation and medication that just added to my list of symptoms.

My primary goal in working with my energy was to experience physical healing. What I experienced was that and so much more. I've seen a remarkable improvement in my blood pressure, my hormones and adrenals are balanced, and I've dramatically shifted my perspective on stress. I used to almost view it as fuel, but no longer.

It's amazing how my approach is now very different. Without stress and without the adrenaline rush, I get a lot more done in a lot less time. The way I go about my work is a lot more meaningful and constructive. I can now see that my employees, clients and I are all working towards a common goal. My work is now much more collaborative.

These improvements excited me so deeply that I sought out other programs that would give me an opportunity to open up the part of myself and my personality that I had closed off, and enable me to really be the vision of the person I want to be as I move forward in my development.

Through the work I've done I have found more meaningful connections in my personal and family relationships, as I'm showing up more authentically. The realisation that the health of my relationships was fundamentally rooted in my relationship with myself has caused a dramatic shift. This work has been very applicable to my day to day life. It's amazing how easy it is to create change if you're conscious about doing it.

Questions

Why have I crashed when I was feeling so great a few days ago?

When you feel really good you open up and receive more energy. It's like a jet hose pouring through your system. Sometimes when you receive that extra energy, it dislodges some older, blocked energy from your body. If that blockage was rather solid because it's been there for a long time, it can be uncomfortable as it's coming out.

How you experience this is that you were feeling really great and now you've crashed. You feel awful. Essentially you're feeling that old stuff coming out. It's like you've had constipation for a long time, but now what's in you has got to come out. This can be uncomfortable, but it's also a time to be grateful that you're clearing out a bit more of the garbage you've accumulated because it's going to make you feel much better in the long term.

Am I trying too hard?

When you need to recharge your energy, especially if you're wound up, it's easy to force it. You try to relax and recharge in the same way that you're used to working. Your inner dialogue runs like this: "I've *got* to relax, I've *got* to get some energy, I've *got* to do it fast and it's *got* to be now." Relaxation becomes just another item on your to do list.

But relaxation and enjoyment can't be forced. They're about allowing. Sometimes it means you have to sit there for a while and wait. It will feel like nothing's happening. You'll feel impatient and that it's a waste of time. Your mind will tell you to do something more useful.

> *Relaxing is not about you doing. It's about you **not** doing it.*

But you need to allow the energy to flow in its own way. Relaxing is not about *you doing*. It's about you *not* doing it. It's about you allowing, receiving, being relaxed. Just being. If you find yourself in a position where you're trying to force things, that's not relaxing. You need to let go and allow it to happen naturally.

The same goes for enjoyment.

Can I relax instead of sleeping when I'm really busy?

Don't get into the habit of trying to use relaxation to avoid sleep and good food. You need to take care of your energy, but you also need to take care of your body.

The extraordinary

Once you master the art of recharging your energy, it's quite remarkable just how much difference it can make.

I've seen busy executives gain three hours of additional productivity every day. I've seen leaders at the peak of the busiest time of their year say they're not stressed because they recharge for just ten minutes at lunchtime. One sales manager told me it was the first time in many years that he had enough energy for his wife and to play with the kids in the evenings.

It's extraordinary how simple this is, if you put a priority on your energy.

Keys to recharge your energy

- Recharging is natural.
- Maintain the charge.
- Recharging creates balance.
- Sleep, relax, take time off.
- Enjoy and be present.
- _____
- _____
- _____
- _____
- _____

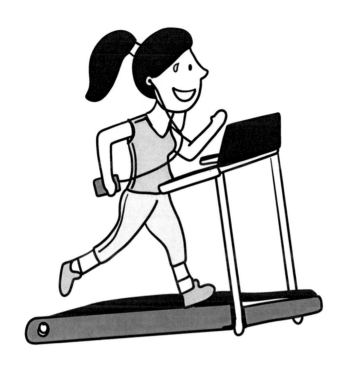

4

Sustain your energy

Sustaining your energy means making energy a part of your lifestyle. Rather than a quick fix that you later forget, it's at the heart of your life every single day, in everything you do.

Sustaining energy is built around habits and self-discipline, so it's actually the opposite of a quick fix. If you take your future success and contribution seriously and want to make a significant difference to other people and the planet – and that includes your own family – you will need to get to grips with it.

Energy is rather like exercise. It maintains your wellbeing, performance, happiness, relationships, money and business. Every part of your life is touched by your energy. Therefore, every part of your life is touched by the way you *care for* your energy.

Sustaining your energy is essential. It is a topic that needs to be discussed in every situation where people struggle with lack of engagement, depression, lack of productivity, poor performance and lack of achievement. These are all energetic problems.

Taking care of your energy in the long term is key to preventing burnout, major diseases and the problems of aging. It's also key to the development of yourself as a human being.

If you fail to sustain your energy you can't keep up the highest level of performance all the time, so it's easy to develop a crash and burn mentality. You throw everything into work when you really need to, and then you either crash or you have to take a whole lot of substances to help you recover so you can start all over again. That's not a successful strategy for life. It can work in the short term, but it's a disaster in the long term.

> *Taking care of your energy in the long term is key to preventing burnout, major diseases and the problems of aging.*

Another response is to slow down and procrastinate. You don't get as much done as you could, which creates frustration. You can learn different techniques to manage your time better, but because you don't have stable energy, you just shift the problem around without solving it.

Procrastination is essentially not having enough energy to get things done. By far the simplest way to solve this problem is to build up your energy. When you have more energy, you're not going to have any desire to leave things undone because it doesn't feel good.

If you fail to sustain your energy over the long term, you become disappointed in yourself because you can feel you're not at your best. You know you have more potential, capacity and capability than you're accessing, which ultimately leads to dissatisfaction, resentment and even depression. That exacerbates the situation because when you're depressed, you have very, very little energy.

If you keep your energy clean, balanced and recharged and keep yourself relaxed so you're not experiencing stress, you build a strong foundation for a life of achievement and happiness. You're protecting your health and enabling yourself to continue contributing well into your later years if you want to.

How to sustain your energy

Sustaining your energy requires you to make lifestyle changes, which actually takes energy. I find that most people who want to change fail simply because they don't have enough energy to take the steps they need to with any consistency.

> *Most people who want to change fail simply because they don't have enough energy to take the steps they need to with any consistency.*

In my experience with many thousands of people over the past 20 years, I've discovered that the key is to learn to relax first, before you tackle your lifestyle. Once you have more energy, many of the lifestyle changes you want to make happen virtually automatically.

You start to exercise because you want to. You clean out your house. You find yourself choosing healthier food. You stop smoking because it no longer feels good. You cut down on alcohol because there's simply no need for it. You feel relaxed. You drink less coffee, wake up earlier and feel more alive.

The real beauty of this is that many of those changes will more or less make themselves. When you have more positive energy in your system, you automatically do more positive things. You don't need lots of willpower. It's a rather simple, automatic way of creating change in your life.

When it comes to lifestyle it's very difficult to make recommendations. I believe that different people need different diets, exercise regimes and other daily habits. This book is not the place for that level of detail, and there are many other books and websites to give you more information. Check out my website for some starting points —www.sarahmccrum.com/resources.

There is also a lot of controversy about healthy lifestyles. I have come across experts recommending you drink one litre of water a day, and others who state that you need six litres. This is a vast variation. And when it comes to diet, the advice is so mixed and confusing that it's impossible to design the ideal diet for anyone given our current state of knowledge.

> *The principle is to love your body. It's easy to go out of your way for something you love.*

So I take a different approach. I will share a principle with you that makes it easier to make any lifestyle change you want and also helps you make decisions about which changes are right for you.

This principle is so simple and powerful that it cuts through almost all the health advice currently crowding the media. It's the only approach I have found that works consistently without causing confusion.

The principle is to love your body.

Your body is a part of life. It's an intrinsic, inseparable, connected part of the entire system of life. Can you imagine treating a small child the way you treat your body? Can you imagine speaking to a small child the way you speak to your body with your inner voice?

What difference would it make if you treated your body with love?

It's very difficult to give instructions on how to love something. Love is part of your DNA and you already know how to do it. Think of someone who loves their car. How much attention and energy do they give their car? How do they look after it? How do they find out how to solve problems with it? You don't need to tell them. They'll willingly go and do the research and find a solution.

The simplest way to come to love your body is by engaging with the idea of it. Ask yourself obvious questions. If you truly loved your body, how would you treat it differently? Is it possible to love your body? What would you need to change to do that?

No one can give you the answers to these questions except for yourself, so you need to ponder them. Let them roll around in your mind and influence you. You know how to love. It's a question of whether you see the value in it. Once you do, you'll naturally find ways to love your body.

Daily movement

If you love your body, you will move daily. Your body wants to move. Your body needs to move. Your body expresses itself through movement.

If you look at young children, they're rarely still unless they're asleep. They roll their joints in every direction, they move upside down and the right way up, they lie down on their backs and kick their legs in the air, they climb and crawl and stretch and wriggle all over the place. They use every muscle in their bodies completely naturally.

If you can allow yourself to explore what it means to love your body, you'll want to take some exercise. You'll start to notice how restless you feel if you sit in meetings all day, or how frustrating it is to be static for too long. You may find yourself wanting to walk or get outside in the fresh air from time to time.

And if you love your body, you'll find a way to listen and respond. It's easy to go out of your way for something you love. Just 30 minutes walking every day makes a significant difference to your health and wellbeing, and can be done in so many different ways.

Try going for a walk when you're having a meeting with someone. They will often be as pleased as you are to have a break from the office. Try doing phone meetings as you walk. You can concentrate just as well. It's quite acceptable these days to do business phone calls from the car, so why not from the park?

Walking will not exercise all your muscles, but it's a great start if you're not used to moving enough. The key here is the love, not the exercise. You will look after something you love. If you don't respect and love your body it doesn't matter how much advice you're given about exercise, you'll end up punishing it or letting it down. But if you love your body, you'll find it much easier to want to move more frequently and naturally.

Water

If you love your body, you'll want to keep it clean on the inside as well as the outside. Drinking water is a physical way of cleaning your body and all its cells. Being dehydrated is unfortunately very common, and it causes many health problems.

There's a lot of conflicting advice about how much water to drink every day, so let's get some principles clear that you can base your habits around.

· Start the day by drinking 1/2 to 1 litre of water (1 litre = 1 US quart). This cleans the entire system.

- Drink plain water during the day (not only tea or coffee).

- Drink a little at a time, not a whole glass at a time (except first thing in the morning when you can drink it all down in one go). This helps to prevent overwhelming the kidneys.

- Don't wait until you're thirsty. Keep hydrating throughout the day.

I personally aim to make sure I drink 2 litres (2 US quarts) of fresh, filtered water a day. This is an easy rule of thumb to start with. If you want to be more precise, you'll need to do some research and decide for yourself what feels right among the hugely contradictory advice available.

Here are some Chinese principles about drinking water which I find sensible. You might like to give some or all of them a try. Avoid drinking anything in the evening after 8.00pm to give your kidneys a rest. Don't drink water with meals, only in between. Avoid iced and cold drinks, even in hot weather, as it protects your kidneys and saves a lot of energy. This is because your body has to warm everything you eat or drink to blood temperature.

Food

If you love your body, you will know or find out what foods to eat. Choosing your food and eating it with love is far more important than the precise details of how much fat it contains, what vitamins are in it or which diet you're on.

My fundamental principle when it comes to diet is to heal your digestive system first, before worrying too much about the food you're eating. If your digestive system is out of balance, whatever you eat is hard to digest. If your system is functioning as it should, it will automatically deal with almost everything that passes down your throat.

When you have good digestion, you naturally choose healthier foods. You don't get sugar cravings. You can't drink much alcohol.

Foods that are full of chemicals or harmful ingredients don't appeal to you. You're attracted to the feeling of an easy, comfortable digestive system and nourishing food.

You heal your digestive system by relaxing every day and keeping your energy balanced and well-charged. I've worked with many people with allergies. Many of them were on very, very restricted diets. Cleaning up their energy cleared out virtually all their allergies, and they often found themselves eating formerly forbidden foods without even realising it, experiencing no symptoms.

Once you have a healthy digestive system, you may want to choose a diet that suits a particular goal. If you're an athlete, you'll choose an athlete's diet. If you want to live a very long life, you'll research anti-aging diets. If you're really high performance and you burn a lot of energy, you're going to find a diet that supplies you with the energy you need.

I believe that one of the major problems we have with food at the moment is we've made almost every food into a scary story about health. We're programming ourselves with the idea that everything we eat, sometimes even including fruits and vegetables, is going to hurt our health in some way. This fear is doing more damage than the food itself.

If you can really love your food, your digestive system, your body and your life, many digestive issues will resolve themselves over time and you will naturally choose healthier food. Somebody who's in love with life doesn't put garbage inside them because it doesn't feel good.

Order

A final step in loving your body is to create order in your life. Have structure in your day – a relaxation practice, daily exercise, daily sleep patterns, daily eating patterns and daily work patterns. Keep your environment clean and tidy, too. All of this supports your health, wellbeing, efficiency, performance and energy.

If you're very creative you may struggle with the concept of structure because it may feel restrictive. But in reality, establishing order will allow you to create more. 'Disorder + creativity' can very quickly become 'resistance + procrastination'.

My Chinese Master used to say, "The sun gets up and goes to sleep on time every day. The birds get up and go to sleep on time every day. What's different about a human being?"

Jan Ashford is the CEO of a non-profit organisation.

There's a lot of change going on in the non-profit sector and this time a year ago I was totally worn out from work. I was burnt out and angry.

I was torn with, "Oh, what's the point of it? Why don't I just go and get another job", or, "Is the fight worth it?" I had no voice. I found it hard to speak up. I felt so much resistance internally as well as externally. I had no capacity to fight my way out of what I saw as the darkness.

One of the first changes I experienced when I started to take care of my energy was that I found my voice and started speaking up. That gave me energy and confidence. It changed all my relationships and my connection with people has changed, especially with members of my board who were causing me to feel very disempowered before.

Today I'm a totally different person and people respond to me very differently. It's far more relaxed and I now have an awareness of opportunities around me that I didn't before because I was so hunkered down. It's made me far more present and responsive and capable of doing work.

Recently work has been really flat out for me, but I haven't noticed it. To some degree I get enjoyment out of it because I can achieve so much. At the moment a number of staff have gone off sick and at the same time I'm doing some high level negotiation about funding, but whereas before this would tense me up and stress me out, things are a lot freer now.

I've got an investment in the outcome but it's not an intense, stressful investment. It's more of an energy focus. It's a totally different head space.

When I think back to all the energy I've wasted in stress, thinking about what could happen and worrying about everything, it's amazing to feel the change.

Questions

Can you just tell me what kind of exercise to do so I can get on and do it?

Nice try. I'm sure that if you're asking this question you're not likely to just get on and do it. You may have been putting it off for years already. Seriously, the best way to get exercising, if you don't do it regularly, is to build up a practice of relaxing every day for a while.

At a certain point you should have enough energy that you'll want to exercise. If not, walk for 30 minutes every day. Once you've been doing this for 60 days (at least), go and find a personal trainer or an expert to advise you on what else to do.

Surely the diet we eat is important?

Yes it is, but I have honestly found that eating because of fear (of putting on weight, getting cancer or eating toxic chemicals) or putting yourself on any kind of rigid diet is almost always short-lived and counterproductive. That's why I am emphasising love rather than food.

It's an almost magical trick to help you find the key to eating well.

Can you drink too much water?

Yes, you can. You can overwhelm the kidneys, which leads to water intoxication. This seems to happen occasionally when people drink six litres a day or more and it is very dangerous.

Get some good guidance from a nutritionist or online medical website if you're not sure how much to drink. I don't give categorical advice about this because there are so many different theories these days and it's not easy to know which are correct. But I am sure that too little water or too much water are dangerous to health.

The ease

Changing your energy is strangely easy. We're so used to life being complicated that it can take time to adjust to this. Every step you take makes a difference and will continue to make a difference for the rest of your life.

If you can have the patience to do the little things and be consistent about them, the bigger things will happen without effort on your part. When you have more energy, it affects far more than how you feel on a day to day basis.

The simple act of taking care of your energy will be reflected in the way people take care of you. You'll gradually notice little signs that life is getting easier and you'll feel more supported and better cared for than before.

Keys to sustain your energy

- Energy is the gateway to change.
- Love your body.
- Love moving.
- Love water.
- Love what you eat.
- Love order.
- _____
- _____
- _____
- _____
- _____

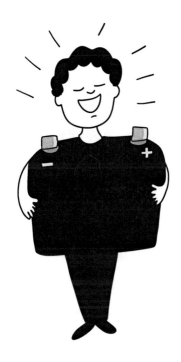

5

Expand your energy

When your energy expands, you expand your capacity. Your capacity is your ability to contribute to life and to the world.

Expansion is natural. You're part of an expanding universe and a system of life that's constantly evolving, so to expand is simply to be who you are in that natural system. This connects with your potential – your sense that there's more you can become.

Being aware of your expanding potential helps you feel on track. You have an inner sense of purpose that leads you forward. You feel more fulfilled on a day to day basis and your life is satisfying even when you know there's a lot more for you to experience and achieve.

Imagine life as a river, with energy as the water flowing in it. You're in a kayak on the river. There are several different ways you can respond.

1. *You paddle upstream.* This is when you work really hard to get somewhere you believe will give you satisfaction and success, but you become exhausted on the way. It's a path of ambition.

2. *You paddle to stay still.* This is when you work really hard to stay in the same place. You never lose control, but you never go anywhere. It's a path of security.

3. *You float downstream.* This is when you relax and let go of controlling anything at all. It's easy, as you don't have to work hard, but you bump into many obstacles on the way and may end up in an eddy. It's a path of going with the flow.

> **When your energy expands, you expand your capacity to contribute to life and to the world.**

4. *You paddle downstream, choosing your direction as you go.* This is when you let the power of life give you momentum and overall direction while you use your free will to determine the path you choose between the obstacles. It's a path of freedom.

So far this book has been helping you to let go of options 1 and 2. The chapter on relaxation taught you how to let go of control and let the river give you momentum. The chapter on balance taught you some basic paddling skills. The chapter on recharging taught you how to recover if you lose your balance. The chapter on sustaining your energy taught you basic fitness and stamina so you can enjoy kayaking.

Now it's time to use your paddling skills as you go downriver. You're probably pretty good at this already. After all, you may have spent years paddling upstream or staying still. But it's different when you're going with the flow instead of against it. Things happen much faster and there's a lot less energy involved. You no longer need to fight the current, but you need to be very alert to where you're going, anticipating obstacles and looking ahead to find the best course.

This is the beginning of the path to freedom, joy and inner peace. It's the only path that can give true satisfaction and deep fulfilment. It's a path of integrity.

How to expand your energy

You need to understand a bit more about how you source energy to be able to expand your capacity.

Think of energy like food. If you eat mouldy food, it will give you no nutrition whatsoever and might make you sick. If you eat junk food, food full of pesticides or old food, you only receive a very modest amount of nutrition. But if you eat fresh, high quality organic food which you cook with love, you take in more nutrition and it's much better for your body.

Energy works in a similar way, but it's food for your life, not just your body. *What you hold in mind* is your food. For example, if you think about an inspiring idea, you're eating inspiration. If you think about bad news, you're eating worry and negativity.

Most people are not aware that the thoughts running through their heads are so powerful. But those thoughts determine the energy you're receiving from moment to moment. They're like programs that create your reality. Imagine for a moment what kind of energy you receive from these different thoughts:

"I love my life."

"Why am I such a loser?"

"I wonder how we could solve that problem."

"I can't stop thinking about that problem."

"This is wonderful."

"This is awful."

"I'm going to win that contract."

"I'm sure I'm going to fail, even though I'm doing everything right."

If you think constantly about problems, you're eating problems. If you nourish your life with problems, what do you get? More problems.

Read the following two paragraphs and see if you can feel the different energy in each of them.

"This is a really difficult problem. I have no idea what to do about it. This is going to destroy my business. This is going to pull everything down. What about the staff? What about the cash flow? What about the customers? I can't handle this. It's too much."

> *The idea is to genuinely love yourself as a human being.*

"Okay, we've got a really serious problem here. I need to find a solution, and it needs to take account of the staff. We have to deal with cash flow, so I need to make sure I bring more cash in as well. How can I do that in time to pay salaries, and how can I make sure we're able to deliver on time so we don't get overwhelmed?"

Can you feel that the energy is lighter in the second example? There's far more energetic nutrition in engaging with solutions than there is in engaging with problems.

This is a subject you can explore for many years, and it's fascinating to see how your thoughts influence your life in ways you may never have imagined. For now I want to share one principle that will help you develop your skill in paddling down the river. It's an expansion of the principle I shared in the last chapter.

The principle is to love yourself.

I'm not talking about being selfish, arrogant or self-satisfied. The idea is to genuinely love yourself as a human being, just as you love the people who are closest to you. When you truly love yourself, you find you also love other people. They go together.

You'll need to explore this over time. I can't give you an instruction manual for how to love yourself. I can simply point you in this direction and tell you why it's worth investigating.

When you love yourself, you don't deny who you really are and what you really want. You listen to yourself with respect and take action on your own behalf, just as you would for another person you love.

A three-step exercise to expand your energy

Here is a great three-step exercise to get you thinking the right way. It takes about 10–15 minutes to do, although you can take longer if you prefer. You'll need to write your answers to the following questions:

> *When you love yourself, you listen to yourself with respect and take action on your own behalf.*

1. *What do I want to experience?*
   Write down everything you want to experience in your life. This can range from feelings to places, professional to personal, short term to far distant long term. It's a bucket list of experiences you'd love to have. Take 3–5 minutes to answer this question.

2. *How do I want to grow?* Write down all the ways in which you'd love to grow as a human being during your life. This may be personally or professionally. Take 3–5 minutes for this question.

3. *What do I want to contribute to the planet?* Write down all the ways in which you'd love to contribute to the planet, again personally and professionally. Nothing is too small or too big. Let your answers flow. Take 3–5 minutes for this.

The point about these questions is that they take you to the heart of what matters most in your life. They connect you with your passion, your vision and the essence of your goals. Answering these questions, and then starting to take action on them, even in little ways, will help you love yourself more and expand your energy. It will put you in touch with who you really are and what you really care about in a very simple way.

Acting on your answers to these questions encourages you to think about a more expanded future, and this attracts expanded energy into your system. It's very different from thinking about "ambitious" goals that you have to push and force yourself to achieve. Those tend to make you tense and contracted, and therefore they deplete your energy, whereas contemplating and acting on these questions energises you naturally.

It's important to stay in touch with your true vision, not forgetting it in the rush of daily business. Find a way to keep these desires front of mind, and remind yourself of them every day. This activates the energy for you to reach them, making it much easier. You may find that some of them happen almost as if by magic, simply because you wrote them down.

Darren Edgell is Technical Sales Director of Smirk Lighting.

It was 'Groundhog Day' with the business. My partner and I were always finding ourselves back at the same place and dealing with the stress. No matter how much work I did, it still wasn't connecting with what I wanted to create. I would overthink things and end up manifesting the problem. Spending my time thinking, 'Oh, we have no work' would bring on just that. Also, I would worry about something that hadn't happened or might never happen, and spend a lot of time going over what had happened. It seemed every year was a struggle and I wanted to change that. I just felt that there had to be an easier way to do business than this. Because I know I don't have the energy to keep on doing it the way I was.

After committing to the practice of relaxation, I have experienced such glorious and profound change in my life. Now, I am able to flip feelings that I previously would have experienced as negative into a more productive experience. Rather than spending my energy blaming others or the situation, I am able to take responsibility for the situation and act effectively.

Business now comes to me that I previously would not have believed was possible. It comes in from places I wouldn't expect. I'm able to identify opportunities that I previously would have let pass me by. By being able to tell a valuable opportunity from a less valuable one, I'm able to use my resources more effectively. My business has gone from working jobs for $3,000–$5,000 to my latest client whose job is worth $600,000.

The energy work has been so useful. Just being aware of where my energy goes. Having those check points, and connecting with like minded people to talk things out so I can check where I am. I've seen the results of isolating myself and not connecting. I just drop down. The more I get out, connect and help people, the better off I am.

Questions

How can I apply this to improving my health?

If you are sick and you want to get healthy, thinking about being sick will make you worse, but thinking about getting healthy will make you better. Thinking about yourself and how miserable you are will make you worse. But thinking about enjoyment and laughing will make you better. Focusing on pain, symptoms and suffering simply create more of the same, so it's important to find any way you can to let go of all that and enjoy yourself more. Relaxation is essential.

How can I apply this to my relationship?

If you're worried about a relationship, personal or business, thinking about what's wrong with it will deplete your energy severely. You can get caught up in this for days, weeks, months and even years, with disastrous consequences. On the other hand, if you simply take some time to think about or write down the good that person brings into your life, to appreciate their good qualities, or to think about them with love rather than criticism, the energy of the relationship immediately begins to shift.

> *Trust that everything is going to be fine. It lifts your energy.*

How can I apply this to money?

If you're worried or afraid about money, regardless of whether you have a lot or a little, your energy supply will become drained and it will become much harder to make money. However justified you feel in being afraid, it only makes things worse, so it's essential to turn this around.

You can't do it by pretending, so you need to find some genuinely positive things to think and feel. You can find ways to appreciate the wealth you have in your life already, regardless of what's missing. A good strategy is to focus on trusting that everything is going to be fine. Trust is remarkably powerful and feels very good, so it lifts your energy. That, in turn, brings you better results. You'll need to practise a lot, especially when your mind wants to freak out and tell you there's nothing to trust.

I feel so stuck in what I'm doing. How can I make sure I actually do some of the things on my list?

Choose something on your list that's reasonably easy to achieve. Make a commitment in your heart, simply by saying to yourself, "I commit to . . ." This is more powerful than it appears at first sight. Don't try to force yourself to do it. That usually makes things worse. Just allow some space in your life, when you can, to take a first step.

I feel so negative at the moment, and knowing this just makes it worse. What can I do?

Start off at the beginning of the day by choosing how you want to experience the day. The simple way to do that is to say quietly to yourself, first thing in the morning, "I want to enjoy today", "I want to be happy today", or "I want to love my work today". This usually helps to improve your experience.

You can use your emotions as a guidance system. If you feel good, you're on track. If you don't feel good, you're off track, so check what you're thinking about. Are you thinking about problems? Are you thinking about something negative? Change it. And be patient with yourself. It takes time to become more positive – and lots of relaxation.

Can I get a quick fix?

Some things will happen more quickly than others. If you relax daily and keep an open mind you will experience many quick fixes along the way.

However if you're looking for a quick fix to reach your dreams nobody can do this for you. You are the only person who can connect with yourself, your heart and your natural desire so that you can find what you want to experience in your life. You will know when you've found it because it will make you feel warm and connected and it will make you smile. There's no hurry and there's no quick fix for the important parts of life.

Why do I experience so much resistance to doing something that I know is good for me?

When you commit to doing something that expands your existence, you will experience feelings of obstruction. It will bring up negative voices in your head, excuses for not taking action, fear and many other versions of resistance. The bigger your commitment is, the more resistance you'll experience.

There's a trick to handling this. Practise listening to the voices in your head that expand you and make you feel good, and learn to tune out the voices that make you feel bad because they contract your energy.

The bad voices say things like, "You can't do that. You're not good enough to do that. You're not worthy to do that. You've never done anything like that before. Why should you be able to do it now?" Not one of those voices makes you feel good.

The good voices that expand you say, "It would be amazing to do that. I'd love to experience that. I wonder how you do it. I wonder what kind of people we need to get that done." These voices open you and make you feel lighter.

One of the biggest arts in life is to learn which voices to listen to and which voices to tune out. Think of your mind as having buttons like those on an old-fashioned analogue radio. You can twist the tuning button to tune into any voice you want and then use the volume button to make it louder or softer. That's where you get to make powerful choices, but it takes lots of practice. Don't get discouraged – keep working at it and you'll see yourself making progress.

I'm totally stuck and I can't see any way out at all. What can I do?

You're stuck between a rock and a hard place. A classic example of this is when you're married and you're dissatisfied with your relationship. If you think of staying in your relationship, it feels disappointing. If you think of leaving, it's terrifying and you don't know if you could find somebody else. So you feel you're completely stuck. You can't change what you've got, and you can't leave it – neither option feels good. It feels as though there's no way out.

The simple principle for all situations like this is to understand that there is a way forward, but you can't see it at the moment. Then you need to trust that it will show up. Sometimes you can gain a different perspective by 'rising above' the situation. Imagine you're looking down on it from above and see if you can discern any solutions. Sometimes you just need to wait patiently for something to show up. Trust is the key.

> *When you wait and trust, knowing a solution is there even if you can't see it yet, you attract the people and situations that can help you find your way out of being stuck.*

To go back to the example of the marriage, I've typically found that people in this situation have no idea that their marriage can be healed or what that involves. Healing a marriage doesn't just patch up the cracks and leave everything the same as it was before. Through healing, the partners gain a new level of love and connectedness they've never experienced before. It's a profound and beautiful experience.

When you wait and trust, knowing a solution is there even if you can't see it yet, you attract the people and situations that can help you find your way out of being stuck. By remaining positive, and not giving into focusing on the problems all the time, you invite solutions.

How can I find out what I really want?

It's vitally important that you connect with what you really want and not what you think you want or what you're supposed to want. If you connect with what somebody else thinks you should want or what you feel you ought to want, there will be no joy in it. You'll remain closed off, and you won't receive any expansive energy. Doing the exercise earlier in this chapter will help you prevent this. It connects you with what you really want deep inside.

How can I get over fear?

If you think small you will never expand your energy. It takes courage to think big and grow. It takes courage not to listen to the voices of resistance. If you don't have a lot of courage, now is your chance to develop it. We all have something that holds us back. Some people have fear. Some people lack confidence. Some people don't have enough energy and others don't have enough knowledge. It doesn't matter.

> *If you're having an uncomfortable time in your life, it means you're expanding.*

You can learn all of it. Take baby steps in the right direction.

Some simple baby steps are to relax when you feel you should be stressed, to trust when you feel there's nothing to trust and to walk towards what you fear, rather than moving away from it. You will find that what you fear grows if you run away from it and recedes if you move in its direction.

How can I see if this is really working?

This process of expansion continues throughout your life. You're going to be expanding all the time, but it usually goes in steps, so it's useful to recognise the signs when a new level is coming up.

It can take many months for a shift to happen, and during those months you may feel quite discombobulated. It can be uncomfortable. Dissatisfaction is always involved, which is a good thing as it helps you define what you want instead of where you are now.

Please recognise that if you're having an uncomfortable time in your life, it means you're expanding. There's a shift going on. If you feel it's been going on for a very long time, you've been resisting the shift. That's why it's so uncomfortable.

The only thing that makes it difficult for us is that we either eat too much rotten food (by thinking constantly about problems) or try too hard and end up forcing everything. The energy lifestyle is about life becoming more enjoyable, more effortless, more easier in yourself, lighter and more natural.

> *The energy lifestyle is about life becoming more enjoyable, more effortless, easier in yourself, lighter and more natural.*

The joy

When you expand your energy, you're on the path to greater joy in your life. As you experience more joy, this expands your energy. A beautiful spiral unfolds over time.

And then you discover one of the most magical aspects of life. When you change, other people change around you. As you open up to joy, people around you who seemed to struggle so much before begin to have an easier time. People you used to try to help or persuade to feel happier start to find their own happiness without you saying anything.

When you give yourself permission to expand, you create space around you for others to expand too.

3 questions that expand your energy

· 1. What do I want to experience?

· 2. How do I want to grow?

· 3. What do I want to contribute to the planet?

· --

· --

· --

· --

· --

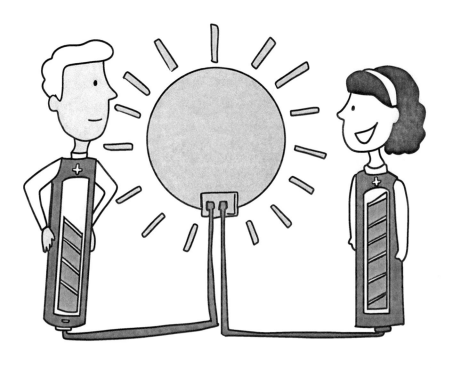

6

Supercharge your energy

When you supercharge your energy, you give it an additional boost that makes life feel even better than everything I've described so far. This isn't about turning you into a human bomb, about to explode into action. It's about giving you access to true power.

What I'm talking about is a subtle and beautiful power that changes you and the people around you with such grace and simplicity that it feels as though it has nothing to do with you at all. It's the ultimate in effortlessness and ease. It makes you feel light, joyful and totally at peace.

This, again, is based on a single principle. The principle is to love life.

When you love life, you live differently. That's what we're going to explore in this chapter.

How to supercharge your energy

When you love somebody or something you feel connected with it. It's a connection that softens and opens you and brings out your greatest self. Love is the opposite of selfishness, personal ambition and greed. With love, you can give more, achieve more and receive more than you can probably imagine.

> *When you supercharge your energy it's about giving you access to true power.*

Love is one of the great human experiences, and it belongs at work as much as it does in the family. It grows through personal exploration, and there's no recipe for it. Love will continue to grow throughout your life if you give it enough space. Above all, it changes you as a person, and it's the only path to your true greatness.

Love grows through connecting. We've already explored ways of loving and connecting with yourself. Now let's look at how you connect with other people, nature and the divine world.

Please forget about efficiency, speed and getting things done for a little while. If this chapter causes you to reflect a little more on your life or ask some deeper questions, you're already on the path. That's enough for now. The answers will show up as you move further along this path of enquiry.

Connect with people

If you love life, you see other people as part of life and you connect with them. You see them as human beings, just like you, each with their unique perspective and greatness. As a leader, you enjoy seeing them grow and develop alongside you, however humble their position in an organisation.

It's challenging if you're not used to working this way, but there's no hurry. This is the important stuff in life. It will give you a deep sense of purpose and fulfilment, so you have the rest of your life to learn and grow.

Here are some good starting points, whether you already have a big heart or you're stepping into new territory that makes you feel very exposed and unsure of yourself.

Take time to listen to people

Ask them open questions about themselves and their lives, and allow yourself to be genuinely interested in what they have to share. To do this, you need to let go of your own agenda, tune out the thoughts running through your mind and listen deeply. Make a point of looking for what's special about them, without comparison or judgement. This will change the dynamic between you.

Practise listening before you speak

This is useful in meetings, teams and any situation where you need to cooperate with others. You may think you already have the answers and solutions, but it's not all about you. Other people need to engage with the answers too. If you always speak first, you'll have to work very hard to bring people with you. If you listen to them, they'll be more willing to come with you.

Appreciate people

Take time to appreciate what another person is contributing to your life – especially anyone you're feeling dissatisfied with.

Write it down, in detail. This is powerful when you're unhappy with a personal relationship or with any close business relationship. It's amazing how much other people are giving you and doing for you, and you may be focusing exclusively on where they're letting you down.

Connect with the natural world

Another way of supercharging your energy based on this principle is to connect with the natural world and experience the symbiotic relationship you have with all of life.

You're part of nature. You're not separate from it. You operate on exactly the same principles that nature does. It's so easy to forget that. When you connect with nature, it balances you and makes you more open.

> *The principle is to love life. Love is the opposite of selfishness. With love, you can give more, achieve more and receive more.*

When you think a lot, you're usually trying to control nature or impose your personal desires on the unruly behaviour of life itself. It's like trying to control a group of three-year-olds. The minute you have one aspect of the situation where you want it, another starts to move and shift.

When you quieten down, and surround yourself with raw nature, it feeds and nurtures your energy. It helps you to come into a right relationship with yourself and all of life. Here are some ways you can connect more deeply with the natural world.

Take some time every day to connect with nature. Go outside, go for a walk, go to the park, spend some time in the garden.

Stop and look around you, wherever you happen to be. Take your time. Don't rush.

Breathe. Take in the fresh air, slowly. Take in the atmosphere.

Feel. Let go of thinking and allow yourself to tune into the pulse of nature. Feel the sun, rain and other elements on your face and body. If you're indoors, feel the ambient temperature on your skin and look out of the window to connect with the weather.

Appreciate. Look for beauty. Look for the extraordinary that's all around you – the flowers, the grass, the insects, the trees. All so easy to take for granted, and yet so unimaginably beautiful.

Be still.

Connect with the divine

The most powerful way of all to supercharge your energy is to connect with the divine aspect of life. Essentially, it means connecting with a presence or existence that is at the source of the visible universe, however you conceive of that. It's greater than anything you can describe or probe with your rational mind.

Something special happens when you do this. It's deeply satisfying and calming to the higher part of yourself. It feels as though everything in life is in order, and it brings inner peace.

When you connect with the divine, you have a direct experience of your purpose in life. You have a sense of who you really are, and you connect with your higher self which is the divine part of you.

This is not *thinking* about who you are, what you're doing here and what life is all about. It's *knowing* it. You *are* it. It's a very profound experience which gives you answers to life's biggest questions.

A divine connection also gives you direct experience of the greatest values in life. These are the values that are universally recognised, like simplicity, beauty, peace, joy, freedom and liberation. All those higher values come from being connected with divine energy, divine consciousness or spirituality.

There are many different ways to do this. Below are two methods that are valuable whether you have a religious affiliation or not and whether you've had previous spiritual experience or not. Both are worth practising frequently. Allow 15 minutes at a minimum for each, and feel free to take longer if you want.

1. Who am I?

Sit very quietly with your eyes closed and relax for a few minutes to calm down. Start to observe yourself internally, as if from the outside. Observe your body and what's happening to it. How is it feeling? How is it reacting? Is there any part of your body that's feeling more strongly than the rest? Are there any unusual sensations? Simply watch, quietly, without judgement for a few minutes.

Now move on to observe your emotions. What's going on emotionally? How are you feeling right now? Remember, you're watching your emotions, not feeling them. Observe them for a few minutes, again without judgement. There's no right or wrong here, just the reality of what you observe.

Then move on to observe your mind and how it's thinking. Avoid getting involved in the thoughts themselves. This is a time to watch them, as if from the outside. Watch how your mind jumps from one thought to the next. Watch how those thoughts flow and move and shift. Let go of any desire to judge them, change them or control them. You are an observer.

For the last few minutes, reflect quietly on the question "Who am I?" Are you the body, emotions and thoughts you were observing? In which case, who is doing the observing? Are you the observer? In which case, who is the body, emotions and thoughts? What's the difference between the observer and the observed?

This is a very deep exploration, and we're just touching the surface here. If you're able to observe your body, mind and emotions, you're taking the first step of realising who you are.

You will discover for yourself that you're not your mind, you're not your body, you're not your thoughts and you're not your feelings. They are things you experience, but they are not the sum total of yourself and they are not your true self. There is another self that is more real and more powerful than the daily, busy you.

2. Experiencing the presence of the divine

Sit quietly with your eyes closed and relax for a few minutes to calm down. Silently, deep inside yourself, ask to feel the presence of God, the Divine, Spirit, the Light, the Source, the Creator, Infinite Being, Ultimate Truth – choose your own terminology. As you ask, you're opening yourself up to feel or become aware of this presence.

Sit very, very quietly and trust whatever you experience. You may feel different, or you may not. It may not be what you expect, so watch out for very subtle shifts in your experience.

Some of the things you could experience include inner calmness, quietness in your mind, a feeling of protection, security or safety, a sense of power or presence in the room with you, tears, an inner melting sensation, a sense that something profound is happening, feeling 'at home', feeling at one, being your true self, feeling very ordinary and natural, or even a feeling that nothing is happening at all. Whatever occurs is just fine – don't judge and don't mentally probe for deep meaning. Simply allow yourself to be with the experience however it unfolds, and trust that it is happening just as it should.

Juliana Edgell is Sales Director of Smirk Lighting and is mother of 3 children.

Previously I thought creating a perfect picture of home was love. So the kids behaved beautifully, they did everything I wanted them to do, we had a calm house at seven thirty, everyone cleaned their teeth, put their pyjamas on and everything was rosy.

But that wasn't happening and my response was feeling frustration, anger, anxiety and hopelessness that I'm not as good as all the other mums out there. The reality was my energy was morphed into the kids' energy so there was no separation between us. It was like a venn diagram where all of the circles were different colours and I was in the middle, trying to blend into all of the colours at once. I felt if the kids weren't happy or they felt stressed or they were throwing tantrums or getting angry with each other, there was a problem.

For me this journey has been about learning to protect my own energy. Now I have a fuller, richer energy in me all of the time. It's like my base energy is higher so my foundations are stronger. Even when something is upsetting or frustrating or I get angry about it, it's never to the depth that it was before.

Now, if the kids are having a difficult time, I say that's just part of their development. It's part of what they have to go through. It's not a reflection of me, it's what's happening for them in that moment. The most powerful thing I can do for them is to be present in that moment.

I now appreciate every stage they're at and who they are in that moment. I appreciate all aspects of them, not just the good bits. So when they're yelling or when they're having a tantrum or when they're running around the house having a fantastic time, it's the same love and connection.

It's different because I no longer feel like I need to contribute to get the love. The love is just there and the kids can't do anything to damage that love. Their poor behaviour doesn't make me not love them and my poor behaviour doesn't make them not love me. There is just love which has changed my energy so much. I feel content and calm just being with them no matter what their mood or behaviour. It's been a much nicer experience for me.

And this extends into my work too. One of the things I've experienced working with men, is that the softer and the more feminine I am, the more effective I am. The more I try to operate like a man, the harder it is because I'm not being me. It sounds really soft and wafty but bringing love to all areas of life, including meetings, brings acceptance, empathy and compassion. All of those elements make for better relationships. You have a lot more tolerance and then you have a better communication platform.

Most people in business want to tell you what they know and they don't care what you know. So they're caught up worrying about making their mark and confirming to themselves who they are and why they are there. Why they're going to walk out of that meeting being more powerful than you are.

The point is, how do you bring love into business? It's just to be present and think about everyone in that meeting, not just about your own intention. If business is going to be enjoyable and valuable then it needs to be beneficial for both parties. It can't just be beneficial for you at the expense of somebody else. I've really seen in my work that I can get everybody to benefit from pushing everybody forward. Essentially it's a basis of love.

Here's a bit about my own experience developing a divine connection, in case it helps you understand the concept a bit better.

In my training with my Chinese Master, we often had to work seven days a week until late in the evening, and I learned how to manage my energy so I never got exhausted. When I was younger I often longed for weekends and holidays so I could get away, but it's been many years now since I've felt that I need a holiday because my energy is pretty balanced most of the time.

Despite this, I reached a point where I realised that there was something missing. I had a feeling there was more to life, but I couldn't put my finger on it. I felt I had much more potential and I wasn't accessing it in the way I wanted, even though I had enough energy. So I started to search for more answers.

It took me a while, but gradually I discovered that there was a different kind of connection, as I've described in this chapter, that had a very special effect on me. It created internal coherence and harmony inside me that made my life much smoother. I stopped sabotaging myself and became more focused and purposeful.

It was obvious that this spiritual connection made the energy I'd been studying for all those years even more powerful. It put me in touch with my true self and gave me an inner stability and security that I hadn't had before.

The way I achieve this connection is very simple. I still often practise the exercises I described above because they are enough. They make me feel more alive and more ordinary at the same time. All the pressure to be someone special disappears. I can be me, and be fully content. It seems like that's all I ever wanted.

Try it and you may well find that the same is true for you.

Questions

I've been practising everything you've said. Why isn't it working any more?

Life is constantly evolving and changing, which means that very often what you've learned previously and what worked for you very well stops working. When this happens, you need to learn something new to achieve the next level. This is something that will continue to happen throughout your life, but it can be very confusing.

For example, you can learn some relaxation techniques, and then find yourself facing a serious challenge only to discover that however you use those relaxation techniques, nothing seems to work. There always comes a point where you just need to let go of everything. You let go of all techniques, everything you know and everything you've learned. You simply go back to the very basics and relax directly. This is the true relaxation at the heart of every specific practice – and beyond them all. It is the ground to which you can return again and again whenever things get tough. You relax, trust and let go.

Can this help me with intimacy?

Here's a small but very powerful tip if you're having problems with intimacy in your personal relationship. Once things get out of balance between two partners it can be very difficult to rebalance. Bad experiences get in the way, nervousness builds up on both sides and blame can quickly set in. Things get worse and a vicious cycle emerges.

> *Love grows through connecting with other people, nature and the divine. It grows through personal exploration.*

Love is the key to shifting this. If you put the emphasis on coming from a place of love, truly 'making love', this dissolves tension and allows for a higher level of experience that can start to break the negative cycle. It's simple and you can do it, but you need to be willing to let go of being right, proving yourself and being the best. Love doesn't score points. It doesn't prove anything but itself. And it gives without expecting anything in return. This will give you lots of energy.

What should I do if I'm an atheist?

When I talk about connecting with the divine, I'm not talking about religion. I'm talking about an experience that's accessible to any human being. If you're an atheist you probably haven't experienced it yet – but the same is true of many non-atheists.

The divine connection is definitely not rational, but it's real, just as love is both intangible and real. It alters the way you think, feel and behave.

If this is unfamiliar territory for you, I recommend you open yourself to a new experience. This transcendent type of connection is one of the great aspects of being human and it's a pity to miss out on that simply because of a label. It requires no special belief, no knowledge and no exclusivity. It's simply a presence you can experience that changes you for the better. It makes you more human and more alive.

Why do I feel as if my life is falling apart?

Essentially, life is a constant process of creating new versions of yourself and letting go of old versions. There's a pattern to this. The beginning of the pattern is that you feel dissatisfied with something and you want more. You want to experience more happiness, a new role, different clients, a better relationship.

If you connect with what you want, instead of what you're dissatisfied with, you connect with the energy of the new version of yourself and you start to feel different immediately.

The tricky part is that this triggers a process of letting go of the old version of yourself. When this occurs, you feel as though you're losing something. In fact, that's exactly what's happening. You're losing an old aspect of yourself so you can let a new aspect in.

The feeling of losing is what makes you feel negative things. You may feel afraid. You may experience terrible doubt about yourself, your life and your decisions. You may feel very out of control. You may even become so uncomfortable that you completely forget the new things you want and start to hold on tightly to what you've got. It's important to be aware of this tendency, because life will become more and more uncomfortable until you let go and allow the new version of yourself in.

The more you recognise the patterns of this process of growth, the easier it is to deal with them when they show up – especially the two difficult parts, when you feel dissatisfied and when you feel you're losing everything.

It's vital to know that dissatisfaction is always the beginning of a new step forward. If you're clear about this, you can say, "I'm dissatisfied. What do I want instead?" That creates a very quick shift.

When you feel life is falling apart you can say, "I feel really negative. I must be letting go of something. That's good. It means there's a new version of me coming that's better." This will instantly neutralise the struggle and make it easier to handle.

My clients often laugh because whenever they're really struggling with something I'm very happy for them and I always tell them it's good. I truly mean it.

> *If in doubt come back to the basics. Relax, let go and trust.*

I have so many questions. How do I find the answers?

If in doubt, always come back to the basics. Relax, let go and trust. The answers will come clear. Sometimes you'll need to be patient and wait a while. Answers come naturally and easily when you relax, let go and trust. It's much more difficult for them to come when you're tense and trying to control everything.

Keep coming back to the basics and they'll support you every step of the way. I haven't found any step yet that I've taken in 27 years where I haven't needed to relax, let go and trust.

The freedom

Something magical happens when you connect at a deeper level with the divine, however you conceive of that. You begin to feel free inside. You may have spent many years looking for freedom in other ways – through wealth, wild behaviour or adrenaline filled activity.

Finally you discover, just as the great teachers have always told us, that freedom is within you. It grows slowly but surely, over years rather than months. Sometimes you can't see it and you feel very trapped in your life, until you discover that your freedom was growing beneath the trapped feelings. It will break through at a certain point. Just relax, let go and trust.

To Supercharge your energy

· Access your true power through love.

· Connect with people, nature and the Divine.

· Relax, let go...and trust.

· _____

· _____

· _____

· _____

· _____

Energy On Demand

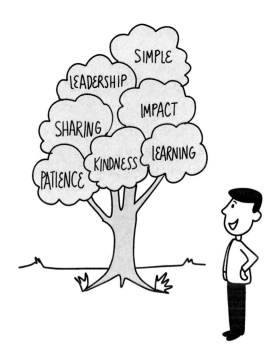

What next?

So how do you sustain all this change in behaviour? The biggest problem you will encounter on this journey to more energy is yourself. There are so many ways you can stop doing the very things that will help you.

You can forget, not have time, feel it's not working, say you'll start again next week, compare yourself with someone else and get confused, find it too slow, find it amazing and still not do it, find it inconvenient, persuade yourself that it doesn't work even when you know it does, decide you're special and need something different and more spectacular, decide you're a loser and nothing will work for you, feel guilty about taking time for yourself, tell fantastic stories about how you know better, tell ridiculous stories about how you know all this anyway, try to rationalise it away . . . I'll let you extend the list.

This is all normal. We all do it. We all need to learn how to deal with ourselves.

There's only one real solution that I've found on this journey. It's to keep coming back every time you get confused or lost. You need to be kind to yourself, forgive yourself for having been confused and have another go.

It's not helpful to give up on something that's important for you just because you didn't do it perfectly the first time. You're learning something you clearly don't know, and that's the most humbling part about it. But there's nothing wrong with a little humility.

So many times I've blamed myself because I felt I should have known better. I had great teachers who told me what I needed to do and I didn't do it. Sometimes I couldn't do it. Sometimes I tried and felt I wasn't good enough. Sometimes I knew I could do it and it would be amazing, but I just didn't. It seemed I wanted to sabotage myself.

But slowly, with patience and the willingness to keep learning, I discovered there was a lot more going on than I could see. I was learning, even during those times when I thought I wasn't. In fact, those periods were often the keys to making a new step forward.

I became softer on myself yet even more determined as a result. I stopped beating myself up, and the increase in energy from this gave me deep inner motivation that I didn't know I had. New experiences opened up that I hadn't even imagined and the rewards started to outweigh the (entirely self-inflicted) 'punishment'.

There is no perfection to strive for, no 100% or top grade you have to achieve and no one who can judge your performance. You're doing this for yourself and yourself alone. It will have an impact on others, but only when you do it for yourself. It's ironic that in being selfish enough to become the best person you can be, you help others more than you ever could by trying to fix them.

I've shared with you six keys to having more energy – how to relax and how to rebalance, recharge, sustain, expand and supercharge your energy. If you only do the first one, and keep going with it, you will change your life and your family, friends and colleagues will benefit as a result. And if you continue working your way through more of the keys, you'll be astounded at what eventually happens to you.

At a certain point in this journey it's natural to want to share what you've learned with other people more directly. You start to imagine what it would be like if everyone in your team had more energy. You wonder what impact it would have if the entire leadership team was putting a priority on their own energy and the energy of the whole business.

You begin to see that lack of energy is a significant contributor to lack of engagement, poor productivity, weak performance and problems with health and wellbeing. In fact, energy work is a much easier way of solving these issues than many other approaches which focus so much on the problems that they tend to exacerbate them.

In my experience, this is a point at which a lot of doubt can arise. I've deliberately taken you on a rather personal journey here, because energy is very personal. It's not just a question of eating the right food and exercising every day. An inner change needs to happen first. Otherwise the outer changes don't tend to stick.

If you imagine introducing this approach to other people, it's easy to worry about those who might not understand, or find it unacceptable. Would they find it too personal? What happens if they don't want to do it? Is it okay to encourage people to relax more, or will they become lazy? What will other people think?

So let's get clear about this. This is a leadership issue. This is where you get to decide whether you take on the challenge of improving productivity, wellbeing and engagement for real.

The great advantage of a personal approach is that it's simply not necessary for everyone to do it. Each individual who improves their personal energy becomes a little beacon, lighting up other people around them. They create energy hotspots that influence the entire organisation, just as you will when you have more energy yourself.

This type of change happens one person at a time. It's deeply personal for each of them, but it's also highly professional in its outcomes, as I've shown through the business-related examples in this book. The change can start with you alone, and you can expand it as gently and slowly as you want. The beauty of it is that a slower, gentler yet more genuine change will be more powerful and long-lasting in the end than a big bang that fizzles out after a few months.

> *So let's get clear about this. This is a leadership issue.*

So I invite you to take your next step on this journey of personal discovery. It might involve starting the 5 Day Energy Charge and sticking to it all the way through. It might be committing to continue relaxing every day for 365 days, once you finish the 5 Day Charge. Or it might be buying a copy of this book for someone else and having a chat with them about it.

As long as it's a simple step, you'll do it. Please remember that. Simplicity works, and it will eventually change your life and the lives of those around you.

Your next steps

- ---
- ---
- ---
- ---
- ---

Energy On Demand

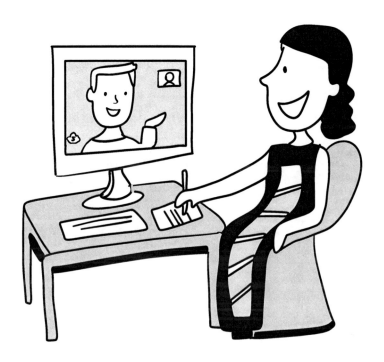

How to work with me

I specialise in teaching CEOs, leaders and their teams how to take care of their personal energy so they never burn out.

You can work with me as a mentor, one on one or in a small group, if you want to create an outstanding personal and business life based on the principles in this book.

You can run a 30 Day Energy Challenge in your organisation to improve energy, engagement, performance, health and wellbeing.

You can organise a group training program for your team to apply the knowledge in this book to help you achieve a specific outcome.

I also create customised programs for organisations to handle specific challenges. These include extreme stress, exhaustion and burnout, depression, chronic pain and management of chronic illness.

Send me an email to start a conversation and explore what you want.

sarah@sarahmccrum.com

www.sarahmccrum.com

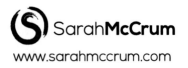
www.sarahmccrum.com

CPSIA information can be obtained
at www.ICGtesting.com
Printed in the USA
LVOW07s0337021116

511251LV00011B/60/P